Katharine Briar-Lawson, PhD
Joan Levy Zlotnik, PhD, ACSW
Editors

Charting the Impacts of University-Child Welfare Collaboration

Charting the Impacts of University-Child Welfare Collaboration has been co-published simultaneously as *Journal of Human Behavior in the Social Environment*, Volume 7, Numbers 1/2 2003.

*Pre-publication
REVIEWS,
COMMENTARIES,
EVALUATIONS . . .*

"**P**RESENTS CLEAR, PRACTICAL EXAMPLES of collaborative efforts to educate competent, well-trained social workers. . . . The strength of this text is the rich examples that are offered: collaborations among schools of social work, BSW programs, states and counties, states and their educational systems, several different disciplines, training systems and the state, planning agencies, and clients and providers. Equally important for educators, the book suggests ways to strengthen the Human Behavior in the Social Environment curricula and the design of relevant curricula in general. One of the most useful chapters presents a specific list of evaluative indicators for university/agency partnerships that are preparing students for public child welfare practice."

Jean K. Quam, PhD, LICSW
*Director and Professor
University of Minnesota
School of Social Work*

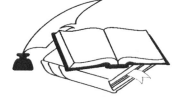

Charting the Impacts of University-Child Welfare Collaboration

Charting the Impacts of University-Child Welfare Collaboration has been co-published simultaneously as *Journal of Human Behavior in the Social Environment*, Volume 7, Numbers 1/2 2003.

The *Journal of Human Behavior in the Social Environment*™ Monographic "Separates"

Below is a list of "separates," which in serials librarianship means a special issue simultaneously published as a special journal issue or double-issue *and* as a "separate" hardbound monograph. (This is a format which we also call a "DocuSerial.")

"Separates" are published because specialized libraries or professionals may wish to purchase a specific thematic issue by itself in a format which can be separately cataloged and shelved, as opposed to purchasing the journal on an on-going basis. Faculty members may also more easily consider a "separate" for classroom adoption.

"Separates" are carefully classified separately with the major book jobbers so that the journal tie-in can be noted on new book order slips to avoid duplicate purchasing.

You may wish to visit Haworth's Website at . . .

http://www.HaworthPress.com

. . . to search our online catalog for complete tables of contents of these separates and related publications.

You may also call 1-800-HAWORTH (outside US/Canada: 607-722-5857), or Fax 1-800-895-0582 (outside US/Canada: 607-771-0012), or e-mail at:

getinfo@haworthpressinc.com

Charting the Impacts of University-Child Welfare Collaboration, edited by Katharine Briar-Lawson, PhD and Joan Levy Zlotnik, PhD, ACSW (Vol. 7, No. 1/2, 2003). *"An excellent comprehensive compilation of Title-IVE collaborations between public child welfare agencies and university settings at both BSW and MSW levels . . ."* **(Rowena Fong, MSW, EdD, Professor of Social Work, The University of Texas at Austin)**

Latino/Hispanic Liaisons and Visions for Human Behavior in the Social Environment, edited by José B. Torres, PhD, MSW, Felix G. Rivera, PhD (Vol. 5, No. 3/4, 2002). *"AN EXCELLENT EXAMPLE OF SCHOLARSHIP BY LATINOS, FOR LATINOS . . . . Quite useful for graduate social work courses in human behavior or social research."* (Carmen Ortiz Hendricks, DSW, Associate Professsor, Hunter College School of Social Work, New York City)

Violence as Seen Through a Prism of Color, edited by Letha A. (Lee) See, PhD (Vol. 4, No. 2/3, 4, 2001). *"Incisive and important. . . . A comprehensive analysis of the way violence affects people of color. Offers important insights. . . . Should be consulted by academics, students, policymakers, and members of the public."* (Dr. James Midgley, Harry and Riva Specht Professor and Dean, School of Social Welfare, University of California at Berkeley)

Psychosocial Aspects of the Asian-American Experience: Diversity Within Diversity, edited by Namkee G. Choi, PhD (Vol. 3, No. 3/4, 2000). *Examines the childhood, adolescence, young adult, and aging stages of Asian Americans to help researchers and practitioners offer better services to this ethnic group. Representing Chinese, Japanese, Filipinos, Koreans, Asian Indians, Vietnamese, Hmong, Cambodians, and native-born Hawaiians, this helpful book will enable you to offer clients relevant services that are appropriate for your clients' ethnic backgrounds, beliefs, and experiences.*

Voices of First Nations People: Human Services Considerations, edited by Hilary N. Weaver, DSW (Vol. 2, No. 1/2, 1999). *"A must read for anyone interested in gaining an insight into the world of Native Americans. . . . I highly recommend it!"* (James Knapp, BS, Executive Director, Native American Community Services of Erie and Niagara Counties, Inc., Buffalo, New York)

Human Behavior in the Social Environment from an African American Perspective, edited by Letha A. (Lee) See, PhD (Vol. 1, No. 2/3, 1998). *"A book of scholarly, convincing, and relevant chapters that provide an African-American perspective on human behavior and the social environment . . . offer[s] new insights about the impact of race on psychosocial development in American society."* (Alphonso W. Haynes, EdD, Professor, School of Social Work, Grand Valley State University, Grand Rapids, Michigan)

Charting the Impacts of University-Child Welfare Collaboration

Katharine Briar-Lawson, PhD
Joan Levy Zlotnik, PhD, ACSW
Editors

Charting the Impacts of University-Child Welfare Collaboration has been co-published simultaneously as *Journal of Human Behavior in the Social Environment*, Volume 7, Numbers 1/2 2003.

The Haworth Social Work Practice Press
An Imprint of
The Haworth Press, Inc.
New York • London • Oxford

Published by

The Haworth Social Work Practice Press, 10 Alice Street, Binghamton, NY 13904-1580 USA

The Haworth Social Work Practice Press is an imprint of The Haworth Press, Inc., 10 Alice Street, Binghamton, NY 13904-1580 USA.

Charting the Impacts of University-Child Welfare Collaboration has been co-published simultaneously as *Journal of Human Behavior in the Social Environment*, Volume 7, Numbers 1/2 2003.

The development, preparation, and publication of this work has been undertaken with great care. However, the publisher, employees, editors, and agents of The Haworth Press and all imprints of The Haworth Press, Inc., including The Haworth Medical Press® and The Pharmaceutical Products Press®, are not responsible for any errors contained herein or for consequences that may ensue from use of materials or information contained in this work. Opinions expressed by the author(s) are not necessarily those of The Haworth Press, Inc.

Cover design by Lora Wiggins.

Library of Congress Cataloging-in-Publication Data

Charting the impacts of university-child welfare collaboration / Katherine Briar-Lawson, PhD, and Joan Levy Zlotnik editors.
    p. cm.
    "Co-published simultaneously as Journal of Human Behavior in the Social Environment, Volume 7, Numbers. 1/2, 2002."
    Includes bibliographical references and index.
    ISBN 0-7890-2034-3 (hard: alk. paper)–ISBN 0-7890-2035-1 (soft: alk. paper)
    1. Child welfare–Study and teaching (Higher) 2. Social Work Education. I. Briar-Lawson, Katharine. II. Zlotnik, Joan Levy. III. Journal of human behavior in the social environment.
HV715.C48 2003
362.7'071'1–dc21   2003001520

Indexing, Abstracting & Website/Internet Coverage

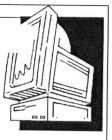

This section provides you with a list of major indexing & abstracting services. That is to say, each service began covering this periodical during the year noted in the right column. Most Websites which are listed below have indicated that they will either post, disseminate, compile, archive, cite or alert their own Website users with research-based content from this work. (This list is as current as the copyright date of this publication.)

Abstracting, Website/Indexing Coverage . . . . Year When Coverage Began

- *Cambridge Scientific Abstracts, Risk Abstracts*
  <www.csa.com> 1998

- *caredata CD: the social & community care database*
  <www.scie.org.uk> 1998

- *Child Development Abstracts & Bibliography*
  (in print & online) <www.okans.edu> 1998

- *CINAHL (Cumulative Index to Nursing & Allied Health*
  Literature), in print, EBSCO, and SilverPlatter, Data-Star,
  and PaperChase. (Support materials include Subject Heading
  List, Database Search Guide, and instructional video)
  <www.cinahl.com> 1998

- *CNPIEC Reference Guide: Chinese National Directory*
  of Foreign Periodicals 1998

- *Criminal Justice Abstracts* 1998

- *e-psyche, LLC <www.e-psyche.net>* 2002

- *Family & Society Studies Worldwide <www.nisc.com>* 1998

- *FIINDEX <www.publist.com>* 1999

(continued)

Special Bibliographic Notes related to special journal issues (separates) and indexing/abstracting:

- indexing/abstracting services in this list will also cover material in any "separate" that is co-published simultaneously with Haworth's special thematic journal issue or DocuSerial. Indexing/abstracting usually covers material at the article/chapter level.
- monographic co-editions are intended for either non-subscribers or libraries which intend to purchase a second copy for their circulating collections.
- monographic co-editions are reported to all jobbers/wholesalers/approval plans. The source journal is listed as the "series" to assist the prevention of duplicate purchasing in the same manner utilized for books-in-series.
- to facilitate user/access services all indexing/abstracting services are encouraged to utilize the co-indexing entry note indicated at the bottom of the first page of each article/chapter/contribution.
- this is intended to assist a library user of any reference tool (whether print, electronic, online, or CD-ROM) to locate the monographic version if the library has purchased this version but not a subscription to the source journal.
- individual articles/chapters in any Haworth publication are also available through the Haworth Document Delivery Service (HDDS).

ABOUT THE EDITORS

Katharine Briar-Lawson, PhD, is Dean of the School of Social Welfare at the University at Albany, State University of New York. Previously, at the University of Utah, she served as Associate Dean for Research and Doctoral Studies and was a co-facilitator of four intermountain west child welfare initiatives. While at the University of Utah, Dr. Briar-Lawson directed the Social Research Institute. Prior to that, she served at Florida International University as Founder and Director of the Institute for Children and Families at Risk. She is a lead author of *Family Centered Policies and Practices: International Implications* and a co-editor of *New Century Child Welfare Practice Servicing Vulnerable Children and Families*. Dr. Briar-Lawson has spearheaded university-community partnerships and family interprofessional collaboration in over 40 states. She has also served as Assistant Secretary for Children, Youth, and Families in the state of Washington.

Joan Levy Zlotnik, PhD, ACSW, has served as Executive Director of the Institute for the Advancement of Social Work Research (IASWR) since September 2000. From 1995-2000 she served as Director of Special Projects and Special Assistant to the Executive Director at the Council on Social Work Education. From 1987-1994, Dr. Zlotnik worked as Staff Director for the Commission on Families and as Government Relations Associate at the National Association of Social Workers. Previously, she held key program development and management positions in child welfare and developmental disabilities in both the private and public sectors. She has served as an adjunct faculty member and field instructor for BSW and MSW programs. For four years she was the editor of Partnerships for Child Welfare, a newsletter that highlighted cross-organizational collaborations and organized several conferences and technical meetings to promote innovation and the diffusion of effective models. She has been a consultant to federal and university projects in this area and has written about child welfare competencies and the links between child welfare and social work. She is the author of more than 18 monographs, technical assistance documents, and scholarly publications.

Charting the Impacts of University-Child Welfare Collaboration

CONTENTS

Introduction

Katharine Briar-Lawson
Joan Levy Zlotnik

Few fields of service command as much public attention as child welfare. When the media bring to light explicit details involving a child who has been badly injured or who died from abuse and neglect, there is a predictable public outcry for change. Cries for change frequently result in reorganizing departments of child welfare, bringing in new administrators, hiring more case workers, funding more foster care providers or developing enhanced parenting, childcare or substance abuse programs.

Workforce development is often a less visible, yet critical response to service delivery crises and efforts to improve child and family outcomes. Workforce development can include the improvement of pre-service and in-service staff training programs, upgrading of the staffing requirements for front-line and supervisory staff, improved supervision strategies, reduced workloads, and enhanced access to resources for workers. When service systems such as child welfare lack a reliable, relevant and competent workforce the consequences can be irreparable. This has been especially apparent given the fact that the child welfare field underwent a de-professionalization phase in the 1970s and 1980s (Pecora et al., 2000). To this day, there are caseworkers in public child welfare who lack a college degree, let alone a degree in social work or in a closely related field.

In New York City, in response to the public outcry and intense scrutiny of the child welfare system after the death of Eliza Izquierdo, the Administration for Children's Services increased its staffing requirement from a bachelor's degree to a bachelor's degree in human services for front-line child welfare

[Haworth co-indexing entry note]: "Introduction." Briar-Lawson, Katharine, and Joan Levy Zlotnik. Co-published simultaneously in *Journal of Human Behavior in the Social Environment* (The Haworth Social Work Practice Press, an imprint of The Haworth Press, Inc.) Vol. 7, No. 1/2, 2003, pp. 1-4; and: *Charting the Impacts of University-Child Welfare Collaboration* (ed: Katharine Briar-Lawson, and Joan Levy Zlotnik) The Haworth Social Work Practice Press, an imprint of The Haworth Press, Inc., 2003, pp. 1-4. Single or multiple copies of this article are available for a fee from The Haworth Document Delivery Service [1-800-HAWORTH, 9:00 a.m. - 5:00 p.m. (EST). E-mail address: getinfo@haworthpressinc.com].

workers. In 1998, in response to a number of child injuries and deaths, the Maryland legislature passed House Bill 1133 which upgraded requirements for child welfare staff and supervisors, creating a stronger requirement for workers with a social work or related degree and also requires the state to develop a child welfare worker certification program. In Illinois, to address the many class action lawsuits that the Illinois Department of Children and Family Services (DCFS) was working under, the Department sought accreditation by the Council on Accreditation for to Children and Family Services. One aspect of meeting accreditation standards required that all supervisors have an MSW or related degree. Thus, DCFS sent over 100 supervisors to MSW programs across the state, enhancing the knowledge and skills of these key staff in the child welfare system.

Over the past two decades, crack-cocaine and correlates such as persistent poverty and unemployment, domestic violence, substance abuse and mental health challenges have swept communities. These risk factors have accelerated child maltreatment and child deaths. In many states they have galvanized the public, media and state legislatures into blaming scenarios. Often overlooked in the concerns raised about the functioning of the child welfare system is the impact that results from the absence of workers educated and trained for the job. High caseloads, rampant staff turnover, class action lawsuits, increasing record keeping demands, and public scrutiny from high profile deaths have in some instances further accelerated the de-professionalization dynamics that have been impeding child welfare systems' capacities to deliver services.

The National Association of Social Workers and the Council on Social Work Education have suggested that just as child safety and family capacity are "public goods" that are to be factored into child welfare service delivery, so should be professionally educated social workers. Over the years the staffing crisis involving high vacancy rates and rapid staff turnover in child welfare provided an opportunity to promote the need for more professionally trained social workers in child welfare. Leaders at the U.S. Children's Bureau, the National Association of Public Child Welfare Administrators (NAPCWA), and the Child Welfare League of America (CWLA) agreed that staffing was a critical issue to address and joined with their social work partners to promote professional social work practice in child welfare.

Thus, in the late 1980s, a campaign was undertaken to rebuild public child welfare systems with trained social workers. This campaign relied on two Social Security funding streams. Title IV-B Section 426 is a discretionary grant program, that has increased from $2 million to $8 million through Congressional action in recent years. Title IV-E training and administrative funds are part of the entitlement program connected to the major source of funding for foster care and adoption assistance. Title IV-E training has an enhanced match and has been an important resource to states in developing partnerships with social work education programs to train current and perspective staff.

At both the pre-professional and professional levels, workforce development has long been a responsibility of schools and departments of social work. Yet partners at county and state levels have also been essential to make the workforce campaign possible. Some of these partners shared the conviction that it was hard to defend having workers with no education in social work serving the most vulnerable children and families. Opportunities are being provided for agency workers to return to school to acquire a social work degree. In addition, a new cohort of social work students at both the BSW and MSW levels are being educated for public child welfare careers.

Several thousand students have been trained using the federally provided IV-E and 426 funds. A 2001 survey on workforce issues conducted by the American Public Human Services Association (APHSA), of which NAPCWA is a major affiliate, CWLA and the Alliance for Children and Families indicated that child welfare agencies indicated that their partnerships with social work education programs are an effective strategy to address recruitment and retention issues <http://www.aphsa.org/>.

Workforce development in child welfare has compelled creative leadership among social work educators and their partnering public child welfare agencies. The benefits of workforce development to the children and families, communities and to the workers themselves must merit the investments. These partnerships have led to experimental and innovative changes in practice, in curricula and in expanding partnerships. This special volume captures some of this milestone work.

Overcoming barriers to recruiting students into public child welfare was no easy task. While many students coming into schools and departments of social work seek to work with children and families, public child welfare was not the preferred job, absent incentives and requisite preparation.

The articles selected for this special collection depict some of the challenges as well as dimensions of these workforce development initiatives. Zlotnik's historical account of IV-E as a pivotal funding source helps to set the stage for the creative approaches undertaken around the country. Pierce provides a snapshot of ways in which BSW programs, producing the vast share of the social work workforce, have joined in to build the public child welfare system. Once funds are invested, are there sustainable benefits? Scannapieco and Connell-Corrick; Chavkin, Brown; Fox, Miller and Barbee all set out to probe retention and return on investment themes.

Preparation challenges educators faced are addressed here. For example, the article by Coleman and Clark probes how the educational program addresses the emotional capacity of graduates for this exacting work. Grossman and McCormick examine effectiveness in interdisciplinary and interprofessional practice.

Collaborative practices, including funding are essential to child welfare especially when families have as many as 14 service providers in their lives, all compel more effective cross-systems work. This is discussed by Phillips, Gregory and Nelson, as well as by Clark and in the article on design teams by Lawson et al. Kivnick, Jefferys and Heier address curricular preparation by examining ways to deliver educational content in such courses as Human Behavior in the Social Environment. Risley-Curtiss charts some of the future challenges in her capstone article.

This collection comprises only a handful of the ongoing evaluative and data driven progress charting involving the child welfare partnerships, now spanning over 43 states. These articles address some of the diverse dimensions of workforce development. They reflect the fact that what began as a campaign for workforce development and reprofessionalization in the mid 1980s has now become a sustainable and even transformational movement.

REFERENCE

Pecora, P., Whittaker, J.K., Maluccio, A.N. & Barth, R.P., (2000). *The Child Welfare Challenge: Policy, Practice & Research* (2nd. Edition). New York, Aldine de Gruyter.

The Use of Title IV-E Training Funds for Social Work Education: An Historical Perspective

Joan Levy Zlotnik

SUMMARY. There is a workforce crisis in child welfare (Alwon & Reitz, 2000). Child welfare agencies throughout the country are challenged to recruit and retain competent child welfare staff to carry out their adoption, family support, foster care, protective service and family preservation programs. Child welfare administrators want to ensure that their current workforce has the necessary training and are also looking for creative strategies to bring new workers into their agencies. Although there is a long history of involvement of professional social workers in the child welfare field, declassification of positions, high caseloads, poor working conditions and a lack of focus on child welfare content within social work education programs led to a distancing between the two. *[Article copies available for a fee from The Haworth Document Delivery Ser-*

Joan Levy Zlotnik, PhD, ACSW, is Executive Director, Institute for the Advancement of Social Work Research, 750 First Street NE, Suite 700, Washington, DC 20002-4241 (E-mail: jzlotnik@naswdc.org).

The author wishes to thank Llewellyn Cornielius, Chair, Donald Fandetti, Stanley Wenocur, Connie Saltz Corley, Diane DePanfilis, and Anita Rosen for their encouragement and support and all of the current and former federal staff whose insights and experiences helped to shape this research.

This paper is based on research carried out for a doctoral dissertation *An Historical Analysis of the Implementation of Federal Policy: A Case Study of Accessing Title IV-E Funds to Support Social Work Education,* completed at the University of Maryland School of Social Work in May 1998.

[Haworth co-indexing entry note]: "The Use of Title IV-E Training Funds for Social Work Education: An Historical Perspective." Zlotnik, Joan Levy. Co-published simultaneously in *Journal of Human Behavior in the Social Environment* (The Haworth Social Work Practice Press, an imprint of The Haworth Press, Inc.) Vol. 7, No. 1/2, 2003, pp. 5-20; and: *Charting the Impacts of University-Child Welfare Collaboration* (ed: Katharine Briar-Lawson, and Joan Levy Zlotnik) The Haworth Social Work Practice Press, an imprint of The Haworth Press, Inc., 2003, pp. 5-20. Single or multiple copies of this article are available for a fee from The Haworth Document Delivery Service [1-800-HAWORTH, 9:00 a.m. - 5:00 p.m. (EST). E-mail address: getinfo@haworthpressinc.com].

5

KEYWORDS. Child welfare, training, federal policy, policy implementation, social work

INTRODUCTION

In recent years, however, there have been new efforts to build collaborations between social work education programs and child welfare agencies to address this workforce crisis. Such collaborative efforts were encouraged through a series of activities spearheaded by the Council on Social Work Education (CSWE), the National Association of Public Child Welfare Administrators (NAPCWA), the Child Welfare League of America (CWLA), and the National Association of Social Workers (NASW), often in partnership with the U.S. Children's Bureau.

In most instances, these new training partnerships between public child welfare agencies and social work education programs have accessed either or both of two major federal funding sources (Title IV-B, Section 426 and Title IV-E) administered by the U.S. Children's Bureau in the Department of Health and Human Services (DHHS) that can be used to support the training of child welfare social workers.

Title IV-B, Section 426 is a discretionary grant created by the 1962 Amendments to the Social Security Act. It provides financial support for undergraduate and graduate education, usually in social work; in-service grants to support short-term training of personnel currently employed by public child welfare agencies; and curriculum development grants (GAO, 1993). Approximately 37 social work education programs received Section 426 grants in 2000 (http://www.acf.dhhs.gov/programs/cb/special/funding/cbfund00.htm).

The second funding stream, Title IV-E, is entitlement funding created by the Child Welfare and Adoption Assistance Act of 1980 (P.L. 96-272) which states may use to train public child welfare staff or those preparing for employment in those agencies (GAO, 1993). P.L. 96-272 specifies that a 75% match is available for "such expenditures as are for the training (including both short- and long-term training at educational institutions through grants to such institutions or by direct financial assistance to students enrolled in such institutions) of personnel employed or preparing for employment by the State agency or by the local agency administering the plan in the political subdivision" (Section 474a, P. L. 96-272). For social work education programs to access Title IV-E funding they must work closely with the state public child welfare agency to develop an agreement and identify the necessary match.

In the Title IV-E program, funds are provided through state child welfare agencies to universities for curriculum development, classroom instruction, field instruction, or any combination of these that is directly related to the child welfare agency's program. Title IV-E provides funds to cover an array of educational supports including: Faculty, stipends or on-going salaries for employees while receiving their degrees, leave costs, replacement staff for employees on educational leave, field work instructors, evaluation of field units and curriculum, program coordinator, educational materials, books, supplies, tuition, travel, and stipends of students being recruited to work in public child welfare services (Schmid et al , 1993). The state must specify how it plans to use these funds in its Child and Family Services Plan which is then approved by the DHHS regional office, must describe planned training activities in its semi-annual Title IV-E claim projections, keep track of the staff trained, and clearly describe the training in the quarterly Title IV-E fund expenditure claim submitted to DHHS (Logan, 1991). No clear regulations specific to Title IV-E training were ever developed and there has been confusion about how to implement this provision (ACYF, 1996; CSWE, 1996; GAO, 1993; Zlotnik, 1997).

Zlotnik and Cornelius (2000) report that, in 1996, 68 programs in 29 states were accessing IV-E funds for BSW and MSW education. Title IV-E training funds have served as a significant resource with estimates of over $50 million dollars currently being collaboratively used in over 40 states to prepare social workers for the challenges of child welfare service delivery. According to Alwon and Reitz (2000), "agencies have seen clear benefits in partnering with educational institutions to aid in hiring workers. To do this, agencies have been creating links with schools that, in turn, send them better applicants" (p. 7). One strategy has been to use Title IV-E funds to pay for employees to obtain an MSW or BSW degree on condition of working for a period of time on completion of the degree. Agencies also use IV-E funds to work with social work education programs to encourage new students toward child welfare careers.

To create successful long-term strategies to build a competent child welfare workforce, it is important to understand the strengths, limitations and history of these funding sources. It is also important to understand the specific targeting of social work education to address recruitment and retention needs. Examining the history of Title IV-E training funding is especially salient, as it has only become widely used since 1990. Its growing use has helped to create new bonds between social work and child welfare. It is unclear, however, why this funding source existed for 10 years before there was large-scale use of it.

History of Title IV-B, Section 426

Title IV-B, Section 426 provides grants to public and nonprofit institutions of higher learning to train individuals to work in the child welfare field. At its inception, and again since the late 1980s, social work education programs have most commonly applied for and received these funds. Through this funding source child welfare traineeships, in-service, and curriculum development grants are available. Traineeship grants provide financial support for undergraduate and graduate education, usually in social work. In-service grants support short-term training of personnel currently employed by public child welfare agencies. Curriculum development grants are used, usually by social work education programs, to create and enhance curricula to teach undergraduate and graduate students the specific knowledge and skills necessary to provide public child welfare services (GAO, 1993).

Funding reached a high of $8,150,000 in 1978 and was cut to $3.8 million in 1982, staying at that level for many years. In 1992 constant dollars, the 1992 appropriation was a 75% reduction from the 1978 funding level, and a far greater reduction from its 1965 inception (GAO, 1993). It remained at approximately that level until 1995 when funding increased to $4.6 million. In 1996 funding was cut to $2 million but an advocacy effort by the newly created Action Network for Social Work Education and Research (ANSWER) restored funding to $4 million for FY 1997 (NASW, 1996). ANSWER is a coalition of the National Association of Social Workers (NASW), the Council on Social Work Education (CSWE), the Association of Baccalaureate Social Work Program Directors (BPD), the National Association of Deans and Directors of Schools of Social Work (NADD) and the Group for the Advancement of Doctoral Education (GADE). (The Social for Social Work Research joined ANSWER in 1999.) Since that time, continued ANSWER advocacy has resulted in increasing the appropriation for Section 426 to $7 million. In FY 2000, the funds are being used to support social work preparation of child welfare workers, child welfare preparation of tribal child welfare workers and training of child welfare front-line staff and administrators. The Children's Bureau annually publishes an announcement identifying the funding priorities for the fiscal year and solicits grant applications from universities, most commonly social work education programs.

Although an important source of training funds for several decades, it has required advocacy on the part of the social work and child welfare communities to ensure that it continues to be funded and that the funds are directed toward needed training programs. Without outside advocacy from these organizations, the program languished without clear direction in the 1980s (Honan, 1985, Zlotnik, 1998). In addition there has not been good follow-up on the outcomes from the funding. The only large-scale examination of the career paths of those who received 426 stipends was carried out by Vinokur-Kaplan (1987). Child welfare trainees from 1979-1981 were followed one year later and the majority of trainees had entered child welfare and over half were employed by public agencies.

The 426 program has served as an important catalyst for innovations in child welfare training and to stimulate the preparation of social work students for child welfare careers. In several instances, since 1990, social work education programs have used 426 grants as a catalyst to seek Title IV-E funding. However, the competitive nature of the grant program, the narrow categories for which applicants are sought each fiscal year, and the limitations of a $7 million annual appropriation restricts its beneficiaries to a small cadre of states and social work education programs.

Background on Title IV-E Training

Since 1990, Title IV-E of the Child Welfare and Adoption Assistance Act of 1980 (P.L. 96-272) has served as the major resource to prepare social work students for child welfare careers. States have worked with individual programs or consortia of BSW and MSW programs to provide degree education for current child welfare staff, to prepare new students for child welfare careers and to provide preserve and in-service training to child welfare staff. The special 75% federal matching funds to states may include university degree education for "personnel employed or preparing for employment by the State agency or by the local agency administering the (Title IV-E) plan" (Section 474A, P.L. 96-272). Title IV-E training funds provide support for current workers to return to social work school to get an MSW degree and provide support to BSW and MSW students who are new to child welfare in order to provide incentives for them to begin their careers in child welfare (Briar et al., 1992).

Title IV-E funds are a valuable tool as states struggle to address their staffing crises and ensure that their staff have the competencies necessary to perform their jobs. As some states and social work education programs began to use Title IV-E funding to prepare students for child welfare work, other states and universities began to learn from them and access this source of funding as well (Harris; 1996). The availability of Title IV-E funds has revitalized the federal investment in social work education (Austin, Antonyappan & Leighninger, 1996; Harris, 1996). Since it only became widely used ten years after initial passage of the legislation, it is important to understand why this happened.

Studying the Implementation of Title IV-E Training Policy

Studying policy implementation brings focus to an important aspect of the policy process which has received little attention by the social work community (Copeland & Wexler, 1995). Such a study helps to understand the political, economic and/or social forces that effect the implementation of policy and which may result in bogging down the implementation of policies.

Since Title IV-E is an entitlement program, which requires partnerships across many levels of government and between government and the university, the implementation process may be more complex than the implementation of legislation, which creates a grant program. Understanding the context which has led to the use of Title IV-E training funds requires the examination of a multiplicity of factors including: the role of social work education in preparing students for child welfare practice; federal leadership regarding child welfare training, especially related to support for social work education for child welfare workers; and the roles of key interest groups in promoting social work education for child welfare workers.

Understanding the implementation of Title IV-E training policy and the extent to which it was intended to be used to provide social work education to child welfare workers, a longitudinal, retrospective case study approach was undertaken. This "single case design with multiple units of analysis" (Yin, 1994) utilized a multi-dimensional framework examining the extent to which the enabling legislation, the policy goals and objectives, federal regulations, clearly defined beneficiary population, role of administrators and their technical competence, agreed upon assumptions, adequacy of resources, organization structure and process, and political issues, are factors in the implementation process. The case study included an extensive review of the literature; interviews with current and former federal staff; Congressional staff, representatives of national organizations and universities involved with social work education and with child welfare policy development in 1980; and analysis of documents including legislation and testimony, federal policy documents, internal memoranda and position papers, newsletters and reports. Chart 1 describes the framework–the factors to be examined, the questions to be asked, the findings and the sources of information used to uncover the history of Title IV-E training policy.

Findings

Vague enabling legislation, vague regulations, variations in interpretation of policy, limited support for requirements that child welfare workers should be professionally trained social workers, lack of leadership in the Children's

CHART 1. Case Study Framework

CONDITIONS FOR POLICY IMPLEMENTATION	EXPLANATORY FACTORS	FINDINGS	DATA COLLECTION
	Clarify the Intent of Title IV-E Training Policy		**Information Sources**
Enabling legislation	Does the statute describe the intended goals and objectives, the implementation process and the implementing institutions? Does the legislation specifically address what types of educational institutions should receive funds? Does the legislation lay out the role of social work education in preparing child welfare workers?	Vague legislative language • Moved from earlier statute • No stated goals and objectives • Does not specifically address social work education	Statute and Conference Report Interview with Congressional staff Memos, if available
Goals and objectives	What were the intended goals and objectives for the Title IV-E program? Were social work education programs perceived to be a resource to be used for the preparation of child welfare staff to meet the goals of P.L. 96-272? Preparation for BSW students to pursue child welfare careers. Preparation of MSW students to pursue child welfare careers. Opportunity for current child welfare workers to return to school to get an MSW degree.	Purpose of overall Title IV-E program is to move children through the foster care system. Other funding streams were intended to be used to support social work education for preparing workers. Training was perceived to be related to Title IV-E goals, not to child welfare broadly.	Literature, published and unpublished reports Review of legislation and report language. Interviews with federal, state and local officials including representatives from social work education. Interviews with interest group representatives

CHART 1 (continued)

CONDITIONS FOR POLICY IMPLEMENTATION	EXPLANATORY FACTORS	FINDINGS	DATA COLLECTION
Federal regulations	Did the Department of Health and Human Services specifically address Title IV-E Training in regulations? Were the regulations developed prior to the implementation of the program? Are the rules and regulations pertaining to Title IV-E clear?	• Regulations for Title IV-E training copied from Title IV-A. (Social work education programs could be assumed eligible because they accessed Title IV-A training funds at the time.) • Regulations finalized July 1982, 18 months after passage. • First set of rules promulgated were very specific. Then a change in the Administration occurred. • Final program rules for Title IV-E were vague.	Review regulations and policy guidance from P.L. 96-272 draft regulations, December. 31, 1980 through *Federal Register* Request for Comments August 21, 1996.
Clearly defined population	Was there a focus on the preparation of social workers to work in child welfare? Is the policy (statute, regulations and/or policy guidance) specific regarding who should be the beneficiaries of the training programs and what entities are intended to provide the training programs?	• Children's Bureau intended preparation of social workers through other funding sources. • First NPRM guided states to use national standards which would require qualified staff. • "State Planning Guidelines" stressed the importance of social workers and need for well trained staff. • Declassification at all levels of government.	Review of literature, policy documents, interest group interviews and interviews with government officials.
	Describe the Policy Implementation Process		
Role and Competence of Federal Officials and Agencies	Who were the key players responsible for implementation at the federal level? Did staff have the technical expertise, time and interest to implement the policy? What is the role of the federal regional offices? Did that staff have the technical expertise, time and interest to implement the policy?	• Many of the key OHDS staff at time of passage were social workers who anticipated that staff delivering child welfare services would be social workers. • Many of the staff were brought into the federal government because of their programmatic expertise. • Training and technical assistance (T/TA) had been planned, but it was not carried out after the change of administrations. • Staff RIFs, declassification, transfer across programs. • Professionalism had gotten a bad name.	Structured interviews with key players at the federal level. Review of memos, policy documents, reports. Interviews with interest groups.

	Clarify the Intent of Title IV-E Training Policy	Information Sources
Agreed upon assumptions	Is there acceptance of the theory that "*Social work is a prerequisite for child welfare practice?*" • Proposed policy supported theory that child welfare workers should be social workers, but little support outside of Children's Bureau. • Policy-makers not supportive. • Little empirical evidence of value of social workers.	Literature, published and unpublished reports. "Review of hearings" testimony, legislation and report language, regulations and policy guidance. Interviews with federal officials. Congressional staff interviews with representatives of key interest groups.
Adequate resources	Are there adequate resources of funding, time and personnel available at each level to implement the policy, including resources for training and technical assistance? • T/TA did not take place because of a prohibition against TA in the Reagan Administration. • New administration philosophy supported the autonomy of states. • Reduction in Force, personnel shortages, personnel turnover. • Loss of institutional memory	Interviews with federal central office and regional staff, review of budget documents. Review of information on technical assistance.
Organization structure and process	• Is there communication between the central office federal level implementers, the regional office implementers and the designated state staff responsible for implementation? • Has training and technical assistance been provided? • Limited communication between central and regional offices and between federal government and states, and states and universities. • Weak regulations. • Infrequent policy issuances.	Interviews with federal central office and regional office staff. Interviews with Congressional staff. Interview with state staff. Review of memos, reports and policy documents. Identification of communication mechanisms and flow between Congressional, federal, regional, state and university stakeholders.

CHART 1 (continued)

CONDITIONS FOR POLICY IMPLEMENTATION	EXPLANATORY FACTORS	FINDINGS	DATA COLLECTION
	• Are there multiple veto points in the implementation process? • What is the structure and processes of the implementing agencies at each level including missions of the agencies involved, and the professional orientation, educational training and previous experience of implementing officials?	• Turnover at all levels. • Technical assistance not provided. • Lack of policy clarity. • Stakeholders unwilling to participate and take risks. • Lack of federal leadership. • Children's Bureau staff with social work expertise lost over time.	Examination of the background, experience and professional orientation and training of key staff at each level. Through interviews and analysis of materials; identify key leaders and social, organizational, political and technical forces or barriers to the implementation of the policy.
	• What are the forces, who are the leaders in pushing for implementation? What are the barriers and inhibitors to implementation? • What is the difference in the support for implementation across time?	• Officials appointed by the Reagan administration not supportive of child welfare programs or social work. • Changes occurred because leaders arose who figured out how to use the policy and diffused the information to others. • Child welfare crisis and lawsuits brought attention to staffing issues. • Confluence of forces: technical know-how, political willingness, class action lawsuits.	Identify differences in the implementation of the policy across time and place through interviews and examination of reports, and other studies.
Political Issues	• What is the impact of changes in administrations, support from interest groups, role of key leaders, and the relationship between federal, state and local governments in the implementation of federally created programs? • Are the bureaucrats at each level, supporters or opponents to the policy? • Is the policy politically feasible? • Are there key leaders who support or facilitate implementation?	• Change in administrations brought a philosophical shift. • Changes in interest groups resulted in little attention to staffing or training issues. • Some bureaucrats supportive, some not. • Policy is feasible. • Reagan Administration policy officials not supportive of social work.	Interviews with Congressional staff, federal staff, state staff, interest group representatives and social work education representatives. Review of reports and policy documents. Identification of key leaders through interviews and analysis of documents.

Bureau, the lack of expertise of federal and state staff, are all interrelated factors that contributed to difficulties in implementation of Title IV-E training policy.

Implementation of P.L. 96-272. A 1980 GAO report, *Increased federal efforts needed to better identify, treat, and prevent child abuse and neglect,* called for a greater federal role in setting standards and supporting training. However, the 1980 election of Ronald Reagan resulted in a decreased federal role and decreased funding focused on training. Prior to Reagan's inauguration DHHS staff had planned to refine staff qualifications for child welfare workers and were supporting improvement of professional training in schools of social work through regional training centers. But the staffing standards were never developed, implementation of P.L. 96-272 was caught in a changing political environment and the focus on the links between social work and child welfare diminished. The Children's Bureau experienced significant staffing cuts and was unable to write necessary regulations, provide technical assistance to help states maximize use of the Title IV-E funding or carry out monitoring visits (GAO, 1993).

The Title IV-E training provision in P.L. 96-272 had been copied from its predecessor IV-A foster care program that had not been administered by the Children's Bureau. At the time of passage, in June 1980, Children's Bureau staff reported being unfamiliar with the Title IV-E training provision. In addition, other more flexible sources were available to support educating social workers for child welfare careers, IV-B Section 426 and Title XX. However, the Reagan Administration brought new approaches to social policy resulting in the end to the Title XX training entitlement, and reduced funding for Title IV-B training. At the same time national organizations shifted their focus away from advocacy for training, as major advocacy efforts focused on saving the larger social programs.

In the early 1990s, as Children's Bureau program staff became aware of the opportunities that Title IV-E training funds could provide, they began to support the use of Title IV-E training funds. However, there were inconsistent interpretations of the regulations among the Children's Bureau and the regional staff. This created confusion because on the one hand the Children's Bureau was advocating use of these funds and on the other hand states and universities were experiencing difficulties accessing the funds. The need for multiple players to be involved in the decisions to use these funds for social work education added to the complexities of implementation. The varying interpretations led to a request for the federal government to clarify Title IV-E training policy. However, in 2000, the policy has yet to be clarified. Differences continue across states and regions regarding how the Title IV-E training regulations are interpreted. The Children's Bureau has been hampered in developing clarifying policy by limited information on whether a policy change would be cost-neutral. For example, if the training policy was interpreted liberally, would higher training costs be offset by lower service costs? Insufficient research is available.

Child welfare crises of the late 1980s. With the identification of the staffing crisis in the late 1980s, key interest groups that had gone their separate ways through the late 1970s and early 1980s came together with a shared agenda–building a competent workforce. Meanwhile, several individuals had realized that the Title IV-E training provision could be used to educate social workers for child welfare careers, and began to tell others. There was a confluence of forces that helped promote use of the Title IV-E training provision. These forces included the focus on maximizing "federal financial participation" in entitlement programs by states, the "staffing crisis" highlighted by NASW and CWLA among others, the need to respond to class action lawsuits brought against child welfare agencies, and concern about competence of staff in meeting the challenges of child welfare agency clients. It often took a new administration in the state and a political issue such as a class action lawsuit or a law requiring licensed social workers in child welfare to stimulate the use of Title IV-E funds. Model partnerships were highlighted and then emulated by others. This is an excellent example of diffusion of innovations. Although the legislative opportunity had been around for several years, it was the communication between the stakeholders that really led to the use of the funding.

Should child welfare workers be social workers? Examining the history of the late 1970s and early 1980s indicates that only a few organizations (NASW and CSWE) and several Children's Bureau staff felt vested in child welfare workers being professionally trained social workers. There was not broad scale support for this within Congress, the administration or the states. With the increasing deprofessionalization of the workforce at the federal, state and local levels, one cannot assume at any level that there is either explicit or implicit support for social work among legislators, child welfare administrators, policy makers or line level staff. Support for child welfare workers to be professionally trained social workers will not come about just based on anecdotal information. Social work needs to show that professional social work education for child welfare workers makes a difference. Without that data, it will be increasingly difficult to target support just to social work education.

Today, there is still limited research beyond studies by Dhooper et al. (1990), Booz-Allen and Hamilton (1987), and Albers, Rittner and Reilly (1993) that specifically address the benefits of child welfare workers being professionally trained social workers. The social work community, including social work educators should be actively involved in research efforts to identify outcomes related to professional social work practice in child welfare. Until there is a larger body of current research that indicates that the delivery of child welfare services can be improved by hiring professionally trained social workers, there will be limited support for bringing more professionally trained social workers into the public child welfare agencies.

Since the decision about how to use Title IV-E training funds is a state decision, social work education should be actively involved in partnering with the state to plan for the use of these funds. Multi-faceted strategies might include degree education for new social workers at the BSW and MSW levels, providing degree education to current child welfare agency staff, in-service training programs, program consultation, staff consultation, program evaluation and program planning. Staffing responses to consent decrees and requiring that public agency staff are professionally licensed are two other vehicles in which advocacy can pay off to support social work in child welfare.

Training is not a given. At the time of the passage of P.L. 96-272, with multiple funding sources available, the key policy implementers assumed that training would occur. With the tightening of funding, and the experiences of cuts to training efforts over the past 17 years, such an assumption can no longer be made. The lack of specific federal leadership on staff training issues in the implementation of the family preservation and support services provisions of P.L. 103-66 in 1993, as well as the passage of the Adoption and Safe Families Act of 1997 (P.L. 105-89) which includes prescriptive administrative requirements without the resources to support the needed training efforts further demonstrate the need for greater advocacy efforts to address training. Champions need to be identified within Congress, the federal government, states and local communities as well as in key national organizations to support such an effort. As a model, the social work community should look back to the creation of the Title XX training program and examine the activism of key social work leaders and their relationships with members of Congress.

Collaboration between Social Work Organizations and Provider Groups. Creation of the Title XX training program in the 1970s as well as in efforts to enhance the use of Title IV-E training funds over the last decade were stimulated through collaborative efforts between the social work organizations and the provider groups such as CWLA, and especially the American Public Human Services Association (APHSA, formerly APWA) and its affiliate, NAPCWA. If the organizations that represent the agencies are not supportive, then it will be harder to garner political support.

Opportunities for Networking and Information Exchange. The opportunities to share information about the use of Title IV-E training funds that occurred through conferences, informal meetings and publications helped fuel the growth in its use. Due to the continued lack of clarity about regulations, the need to share outcome data, the changing political environment, the changing leadership in states, universities and federal agencies, and state and federal staff turnover (resulting in loss of institutional memory)–there is a continued need to provide avenues for such exchange. CSWE can provide opportunities for exchange through the Annual Program Meeting and through its publications. NASW can also provide such opportunities at its state level, regional and national meetings. The Children's Bureau has also assisted through the 2000 *Child Welfare Training Partnerships for the 21st Century Workforce* conference. Support for such conferences as well as continuation of the "Partnerships for Child Welfare" newsletter are important for information exchange.

Since Title IV-E training funds are not federally administered grants to social work education programs, there are no required "grantees meetings" that would be a natural place to exchange ideas. Therefore it is incumbent on the field itself to create opportunities. Programs receiving 426 funds could be encouraged to provide a national forum, as was supported with Children's Bureau funds in the final year of a grant to Southern Illinois University in 1996.

CONCLUSION

Multiple forces converged to help social work education programs access Title IV-E funding. The policy was there, relatively unnoticed and not very clearly articulated. Figuring out how it might be used and telling people about it became important as states and social work education programs sought ways to ensure a more competent child welfare workforce. The initial plans to implement P.L. 96-272 had also intended to encourage a better-trained workforce. The use of two funding sources were anticipated to be used, one that the federal government targeted to social work education programs, and the other was targeted to states who would then contract with social work education or other university programs for staff training. That effort got derailed by a change in the federal administration that brought in a different philosophy–no encouragement of federal leadership, guidance or technical assistance and continual declassification. States were on their own to figure out what they should do, and the staff at the federal level who were invested in helping states were stifled in their actions. What occurred instead of all the hopes of P.L. 96-272 was a system in crisis by the late 1980s. That crisis continues today.

Accessing Title IV-E training funding alone is not the answer to the child welfare crisis. The need for better trained staff has encouraged states and universities to work together to access this complex and confusing funding source. With the limitations on other child welfare training funding resources, it is time for the federal Title IV-E policy to be clarified and broadened, as was proposed in the draft Notice of Proposed Rule-Making prepared in 1993, to meet the training needs of child welfare agency staff. The findings suggests that in order to obtain or maintain federal support for social work education there is an on-going need to study policy implementation; to understand the differences between entitlement and grant programs; to develop partnerships with states; to develop outcome data about the "difference" professionally trained social workers can make; to be familiar with all aspects of legislation; to create advocacy collaboratives that extend beyond the social work education community and to provide opportunities for networking and information exchange.

Do our most vulnerable children deserve any less?

REFERENCES

Administration for Children, Youth and Families. (1996, August 21). Comments concerning the implementation and management of child welfare training for which federal financial participation (FFP) is available. *Federal Register*, *61*(163) p. 43250.

Albers, E., Reilly, T., & Rittner, B. (1993). Children in foster care: Possible factors affecting permanency planning. *Child and Adolescent Social Work Journal, 10*(4), 329-341.

Alwon, R. & Reitz, A. (2000). *The workforce crisis in child welfare.* Washington, DC: CWLA Press.

Austin, M., Antonyappan, J., Leighninger, L. (1996). Federal support for social work education: Section 707 of the 1967 Social Security Amendments. *Social Service Review, 70*(1) 83-97.

Booz-Allen & Hamilton. (1987). *The Maryland social services job analysis and personnel qualifications study.* Baltimore, MD: Maryland Department of Human Resources.

Briar, K., Hansen, V. & Harris, N. (Eds.). (1992). *New partnerships: Proceedings from the National Public Child Welfare Symposium.* Miami, FL: Florida International University.

Copeland, V. C & Wexler, S. (1995). Policy implementation in social welfare: A framework for analysis. *Journal of Sociology and Social Welfare,* 51-69.

Council on Social Work Education. (1996). Social work education programs are urged to provide comments to the department of health and human services regarding Title IV-E training: Action needed by October 21, 1996.

Dhooper, S.S., Royse, D.D., & Wolfe, L.C. (1990). Does social work education make a difference. *Social Work, 35*(1), 57-61.

General Accounting Office. (1993). *Federal policy on Title IV-E share of training costs.* Washington, DC: Author.

General Accounting Office (1980). *Increased federal efforts needed to better identify, treat, and prevent child abuse and neglect.* Washington, DC: Author.

Harris, N. (1996). *Social work education and public human services partnerships: A technical assistance document.* Alexandria, VA: Council on Social Work Education.

Honan, A. (1985). *The impact of interest groups on federal funding for social work education; 1948-1983.* Doctoral Dissertation, Columbia University School of Social Work.

Logan, J. (1991). Federal funding for child welfare training programs, P.L. 96-272, Adoption Assistance and Child Welfare Act of 1980. Briefing paper by Jean Logan, Jean S. Logan Management Group, N. Miami, Beach, FL.

National Association of Social Workers. (1996, May 8). FY 1997 appropriations for Title IV-B child welfare training. (Government Relations Alert). Washington, DC: Author.

Schmid, D., Briar, K., Harris, N., & Logan, J. (1993, February). Creating an interdependent services and training financing strategy. *Partnership Newsletter.* Miami, FL: Florida International University Department of Social Work, Institute for Children and Families at Risk.

Vinokur-Kaplan, D. (1987). Where did they go? A national follow-up of child welfare trainees. *Child Welfare, 66*(5), 411-421.

Zlotnik, J. (1997a). Social work education programs, state child welfare agencies comment on Title IV-E regulations. *Social Work Education Reporter, 45*(1), 6.

Zlotnik, J. L. & Cornelius, L. (2000). Preparing Social Work Students for Child Welfare Careers: The Use of Title IV-E Training Funds in Social Work Education. *Journal of Baccalaureate Social Work, 5*(2), 1-14.

Use of Title IV-E Funding in BSW Programs

Lois Pierce

SUMMARY. Title IV-E provides resources that allow social work education and state child welfare agencies to collaborate to provide an educational experience that prepares students to move quickly into a complex practice experience. In 1998-1999 all BSW programs that were accredited and in candidacy were surveyed to see if they were using Title IV-E funds to provide support for students who would agree to work in public child welfare programs after graduation. The questionnaire used was based on Zlotnik's earlier survey (Zlotnik & Cornelius, 2000) of all programs receiving IV-E funds. Of the 464 BSW programs surveyed, 282 replied, 59% of these were public institutions, the rest private. Forty-eight schools reported receiving some type of IV-E funding for students. Results indicate a number of models are used to support collaboration between the schools and their state agencies. These include differences in the requirements of students while they are in school and after graduation and in the amount of funding available to students. In addition, institutions not receiving IV-E funds were asked to describe why they were not. Implications for BSW programs are discussed. *[Article copies available for a fee from The Haworth Document Delivery Service: 1-800-HAWORTH. E-mail address: <getinfo@haworthpressinc.com> Website: <http://www.HaworthPress. com> © 2003 by The Haworth Press, Inc. All rights reserved.]*

Lois Pierce, PhD, is affiliated with the University of Missouri-St. Louis, 8001 Natural Bridge Road, St. Louis, MO 63121 (E-mail: piercel@umsl.edu).

[Haworth co-indexing entry note]: "Use of Title IV-E Funding in BSW Programs." Pierce, Lois. Co-published simultaneously in *Journal of Human Behavior in the Social Environment* (The Haworth Social Work Practice Press, an imprint of The Haworth Press, Inc.) Vol. 7, No. 1/2, 2003, pp. 21-33; and: *Charting the Impacts of University-Child Welfare Collaboration* (ed: Katharine Briar-Lawson, and Joan Levy Zlotnik) The Haworth Social Work Practice Press, an imprint of The Haworth Press, Inc., 2003, pp. 21-33. Single or multiple copies of this article are available for a fee from The Haworth Document Delivery Service [1-800-HAWORTH, 9:00 a.m. - 5:00 p.m. (EST). E-mail address: getinfo@haworthpressinc.com].

KEYWORDS. Child welfare, Title IV-E funding, BSW education

The increasing number of children and families receiving child welfare services during the past several decades has increased the need for social work programs to prepare graduates for the cases they will encounter in child welfare practice (Costin, Karger & Stoesz, 1996; Zlotnik, 1997). Workers today must address a wide range of issues in a rapidly changing context. The implementation of the Adoption and Safe Families Act has required agencies to develop new policies and procedures for addressing family problems within short timelines. Because children and families with the fewest problems are now reunited fairly quickly, child welfare workers often face caseloads of the most complex and difficult families. Workers must be able to understand how to address substance abuse and family violence. Both of these issues are closely related to child maltreatment, and neither is likely to be resolved with short-term intervention (Smith, 2001; Hilbert, 2001).

In addition to difficult cases and changing policy, workers must be willing to make home visits in some of the more dangerous areas of a city or county, many times with families known for their violent behavior. Even with a police escort, workers must be skilled in defusing potentially dangerous situations.

Pecora, Briar and Zlotnik (1989) and Zlotnik and Cornelius (2000) suggest that these factors of high numbers of difficult cases, unrewarding work situations and changing work contexts have led to difficulty in recruiting and retaining child welfare workers. Anecdotal reports describe workers going out on their first home visit and quitting instead of returning to the office. Workers are often unprepared for the work they are expected to perform and if they don't quit immediately, they often don't last very long. Turnover has been as high as 40% in a Midwest child protection services agency that the author works with (J. Washek, personal communication, March 7, 2000).

One response to recruiting and retaining child welfare workers has been collaboration between social work education and state child welfare agencies. Several studies have shown that graduates of social work programs not only perceive themselves to be better prepared to deliver services than graduates of other programs (e.g., Lieberman, Hornby & Russell, 1988), but also are better at delivering services than others (Albers, Reilly & Rittner, 1993; Dhooper, Royse, & Wolfe, 1990.) Furthermore, graduates of social work programs appear to have lower turnover rates (Russell, 1987; Vinokur-Kaplan, 1991).

Workers with a social work degree were found to be more effective with children in foster care than were other workers (Albers et al., 1993). Children who remained in foster care for longer than three years were less likely to have a worker who had a social work degree. Dhooper, Royse, and Wolfe (1990) found that state agency employees with BSWs or MSWs scored higher than those without those degrees in all areas they examined. Although few studies have examined turnover rates, Russell (1987) found that states with more stringent requirements for employment (i.e. BSWs and MSWs) had lower turnover rates. States lost fewer workers when they collaborated with universities, provided incentives to workers and engaged in retention activities.

Although there is support for the use of social work education to improve the knowledge and skills of child welfare workers and to increase retention rates of workers once they enter child welfare, disagreement continues about what level of social work education is most appropriate for child welfare work. Olsen and Holmes (1982) found some differences in educational levels and effectiveness. MSW workers were more effective in adoption services; BSW workers were better at delivering day treatment, providing services related to mental health, finding employment and financial assistance. Otherwise educational background had little affect on job performance. The findings suggest that BSW workers can be effective in performing most child welfare tasks.

SUPPORT FOR SOCIAL WORK EDUCATION AND STATE AGENCY COLLABORATION

One of the best known programs for the support of collaboration between social work education and state child welfare agencies is Title IV-E, created through the Child Welfare and Adoption Assistance Act (Public Law 96-272). Title IV-E is now being used to train public child welfare staff or those preparing for employment in those agencies (Zlotnik, 1998). Title IV-E funds can be used by social work programs to develop pre-service or in-service training as well as degree programs. State agencies found that when they hire graduates of social work programs with child welfare content incorporated into their curriculum and support field placements in child welfare agencies, workers are able to "hit the ground running" and are more likely to stay (M. Mica, personal communication, June 20, 2000).

Title IV-E funding is for public social work programs, although some private institutions have been able to subcontract with public programs. Otherwise, private social work programs must provide a cash match rather than the in-kind match allowed public programs. Additionally, states determine which institutions receive the funding. A state may use only MSWs for child welfare positions and not fund BSW slots or may decide to fund BSW education.

BACKGROUND OF THE CURRENT SURVEY

In 1996, the Association of Baccalaureate Program Directors formed a committee on child welfare advocacy. This grew out of the organization's con-

cern that even though much of the funding for child welfare education was going to MSW programs, BSW prepared social workers were trained in the
competencies needed to be effective child welfare practitioners. Although
some states limit child welfare workers to those who have an MSW, many
states' educational requirement for public child welfare work is a baccalaureate degree. The committee sought to find out how many BSW programs were
using Title IV-E funds and use that information to help others learn about
funding sources. There was also a desire to provide a venue for sharing ideas
about Title IV-E programs and learning from others' experiences. Committee
members decided to identify those who received Title IV-E funds through a
survey of all accredited baccalaureate social work programs.

Zlotnik's (Zlotnik & Cornelius, 2000) survey of all accredited social work
programs in the U.S., which requested information on Title IV-E funding,
found that 24 BSW programs, 33 MSW programs and 11 joint programs had
Title IV-E training programs. Zlotnik's questionnaire was used as a starting
point for the new survey. Questions were asked and revised based on responses
to the original survey.

METHODOLOGY

In 1999, all undergraduate social work programs listed in the Council on
Social Work Education's registry of accredited programs was sent a questionnaire. Although respondents were told they did not have to provide their name,
the forms were coded so a second mailing could be sent to those programs that
did not respond to the first. Of the 464 schools that were sent a questionnaire,
responses were eventually received from 282 programs, which was a 61% response rate.

SAMPLE

Of the programs that responded, 115 (44%) identified themselves as a BSW
program in a public university, 40 (15%) were a joint BSW/MSW program in a
public university, 92 (36%) were a BSW program in a private university, and 12
(5%) were a joint BSW/MSW program in a private university (see Figure 1).

Ninety-one (35%) of the schools had between 25 and 75 social work majors, 65 (25%) had between 75 and 125 majors, 36 (14%) had between 125 and
175 majors, 54 (21%) had more than 175 majors and the rest had fewer than 10
majors (14, 5%) (see Figure 2).

Responses were received from 44 states (see Table 1).

FIGURE 1. Type of BSW Program

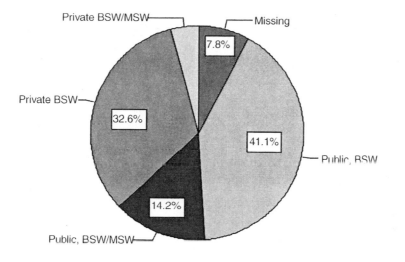

FIGURE 2. Number of Majors in Reporting BSW Programs

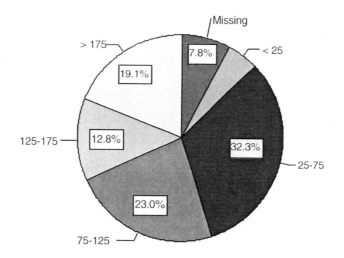

TABLE 1. Responses by States Indicating Title IV-E Funding for BSW Programs and State Model, 1999

STATE	FUNDING	MODEL
Alabama	yes	
Alaska	yes	consortium
Arkansas	yes	consortium
Arizona	no	
California	not for BSW, except LA county	
Colorado	yes	statewide
Connecticut	no, working on	
Florida	no, other funding	
Georgia	yes	statewide
Idaho	no	
Illinois	not for BSW, working on	
Indiana	no	
Iowa	start this year	
Kansas	some	privatized
Kentucky	yes	consortium
Louisiana	yes	statewide
Maine	yes	
Maryland	not for BSW	
Massachusetts	no	
Michigan	not for BSW	
Minnesota	subcontract from U of Minnesota	
Mississippi	not for BSW	
Missouri	yes	statewide
Montana	no	forming consortium with Eastern WA
Nevada	yes	statewide
New Jersey	none reported	
New Mexico	yes	statewide
New York	yes	
North Carolina	yes	2 schools now, consortium starting
North Dakota	no	
South Carolina	no	
South Dakota	no, university overhead too much	
Ohio	no, difficulty arranging	
Oklahoma	yes	administered through OU
Oregon	no	
Pennsylvania	not for BSW	
Tennessee	no	
Texas	yes	regional consortia
Utah	no	
Vermont	yes	but focus on MSW
Virginia	yes	state wide
Washington	yes	
West Virginia	yes	consortium
Wisconsin	no, BSW programs do employee training	

RESULTS

Of the schools that responded, 48 received Title IV-E funding for BSW students who agreed to work in child welfare after graduation. (The questionnaire specifically asked for information on educational funds for students who were working on a BSW degree.) Some programs also received funding for MSW students, but only the BSW program was considered.

Program directors were asked if they included child welfare content in the curriculum. About one-fourth of the programs include content in required courses. Fifteen percent said they had child welfare courses as electives. Only 4 percent required child welfare courses for all students. Another 20 percent had combinations of the above, with about half requiring child welfare courses for trainees and offering elective courses for the rest of their students. The rest of the programs (34%) indicated they did not include child welfare content in their courses. Because the Council on Social Work Education accreditation standards emphasize generalist practice for BSW programs (CSWE, 1994), directors are sometimes hesitant to offer a sequence of courses which may appear to be a specialization.

Descriptions of IV-E Programs

The average length of time that programs had been receiving IV-E funds was four years. Six programs had received funds for seven or more years, 16 programs were in their first two years. The short length of time most programs have been involved in IV-E makes it somewhat difficult to evaluate how effective the program has been.

The number of trainees per year ranged from 1 to 30. The program with 30 trainees provides employees for a large portion of the state. The median number of trainees per year was 5 students.

Stipends provided to students for an academic year ranged from $2000 at one program to $14,000 at another. The mean amount was $5250 and is based on the responses from 45 programs. Although many programs allow students to use the stipends for whatever expenses they have, eight schools included tuition in the stipend. Georgia only paid for tuition, fees and books. Funds for tuition ranged from $1100 to $9580, with a mean of $3900.

Programs were also asked how many of their IV-E students were already working in public child welfare. Twenty-eight programs (61%) said none; one program said 100 percent (14 trainees). On average, 14 percent of the IV-E students were already working in child welfare.

Student Selection and Other Features of Title IV-E Degree Programs

In 75 percent of the programs students are selected for the IV-E stipends through joint interviews with university faculty and agency staff. In some cases the university interviews first, then sends students on to the agency for an interview. In others, they interview together. Faculty select participants in 6 programs (12%) and agencies do the selection in four (8%) of the programs. In most cases agencies use this interview as the job interview and waive a second interview after graduation.

Other special provisions for IV-E graduates include waiving a merit test (21%) and waiving special training after graduation (24%).

Only six programs said they had subcontracts with private universities or colleges; three of these had contracts with one private program, three with two. Eight programs taught IV-E students through distance learning programs, with four of these having one site, one having two, one having four and one having six. One program did not indicate how many sites. Six of the seven sites were in rural areas.

Requirements of Students Receiving Title IV-E Education Funding

Title IV-E requirements vary a great deal from state to state, but in each case the requirements are determined by the state and students sign a contract with the state before they receive funding. The length of time in which students must find a state agency child welfare position after graduation ranges from two weeks to two years. The majority of programs reported their students had two months (44%) or three months (19%) to find a job. Although a few states required graduates to work 8 or 9 months as payback for the stipends, most required either one year (36%) or 18 months (14%). Four schools (10%) required IV-E graduates to work 24 months.

Some states (56% of the programs responding) require IV-E graduates to work in a certain location (e.g., in rural areas, in the county in which they did their practicum, within a 50 mile radius of their home county). Others have no requirements. One respondent said the need in their state for BSW trained child welfare workers was great and their graduates never had problems finding a position.

Thirty-one schools (65%) listed conditions under which IV-E trainees would have to pay back their stipends. For one school, students who dropped out of school or did not graduate had to pay the state back. Fifteen schools (31%) said students had to pay back the state if after graduation they decided not to work in children's services. Another 15 schools said students were required to pay back tuition when they broke their contract with the state. In most cases this either meant they did not work for the state or they did not work the time required for the pay back. States often will work with graduates, extending the time of the contract to allow students time off for pregnancies or family emergencies.

Respondents were asked the conditions under which students would be allowed to be released from their contract. Fifty-four percent of the programs allowed students two to three months to find a position. If nothing was available by the end of that period, they could be released from paying back their stipend. This rarely happens though.

Although the question was somewhat ambiguous, schools were asked if their IV-E graduates could immediately enter an MSW program and postpone fulfilling their undergraduate contract. This was rarely allowed. States prefer to have students with several years of experience before beginning an MSW program, particularly if having an MSW means the employee will work in a supervisory position. In one state, IV-E graduates are able to work for the state and attend an MSW program part time immediately after receiving a BSW degree.

Models

Because IV-E funds are passed through the state child welfare office to a social work program, states have developed a number of models for working with social work programs. Respondents from Alaska, Arkansas, Kentucky, and Tennessee described state-wide consortia in which all of the participating schools in that state work together to provide child welfare education for students who qualify for IV-E funding. In Kentucky, for example, the 7 participating schools have developed one syllabus that is used for the child welfare course. The state agency works with the schools on their curriculum to assure that program graduates all have essentially the same knowledge base and skills. Because Texas is so large, it has regional consortia with schools from each region working with the regional child welfare office to develop a training program for that part of the state.

Other states have worked out programs with individual schools in the state. Generally these schools respond to the state's request to provide IV-E educational services and the schools negotiate a contract with the state describing how they will provide these services. Based on responses, these states include Colorado, Georgia, Louisiana, Maine, Missouri, Nevada, New Mexico, Oklahoma, Virginia and Washington. In Missouri, a state agency staff member coordinates the seven state university programs. One program has students in block placements and uses county-level staff as faculty coordinators. Another has hired a former supervisor who serves as the liaison between the university and the agency, supervises the students trainees' learning experience and teaches a child welfare seminar. Because she knows staff at county agencies, she is able to mediate student-staff misunderstandings.

At the time of the survey, Montana was working with Eastern Washington State University to form a consortium. Other states were planning to implement Title IV-E funding for BSW students. These include Illinois, Iowa and North Carolina. Some states have provided Title IV-E funding only to MSW programs including California, Illinois (which is changing), Maryland, Michigan, Mississippi and Pennsylvania. One exception to MSW only funding in California has been an arrangement in which California State-Long Beach works with Los Angeles County to provide stipends for BSW students.

In Kansas, child welfare training was privatized several years ago, but recently the University of Kansas has been receiving Title IV-E funds again for training. In Vermont, the focus has been on training MSWs, but occasionally a BSW student will receive Title IV-E funds.

WHY SCHOOLS DON'T APPLY FOR TITLE IV-E FUNDS

Most of the private social work programs were aware that they could not apply for funds. Smaller public social work programs frequently said they did not have the time or resources to apply for grants. Many said high teaching loads did not allow faculty to take on additional responsibilities. Several misunderstood the purpose of the funding. One program director assumed the funds were for minority students.

In several states, schools had been working for several years to try to develop Title IV-E contracts with their state agency but had been unable to do so. Some respondents said they were unable to compete with large universities that already had IV-E grants. One respondent suggested that large universities were unwilling to share with smaller schools. Several respondents said the application was too complicated and they had stopped trying to apply. However, a number of respondents said they had not had a chance to look into IV-E funding and would like more information.

DISCUSSION

BSW programs that have Title IV-E funding appear to be educating a cadre of students who will be well prepared for child welfare practice. The majority of students take specialized child welfare content that helps them relate what they are learning in their courses to their child welfare practicum. Students benefit by receiving stipends that can help offset educational fees. They are assured of a job at graduation if they satisfactorily complete their practicum and course work. Agencies benefit by having new workers who know what to expect and have a good idea of the types of families and problems they will be working with. This should provide agencies with workers who are more satisfied with their jobs, more comfortable working with children and families in their communities and more likely to stay with the agency.

Several problems still remain. Because many Title IV-E programs are relatively new, few have been able to demonstrate the effectiveness of their program. Southwest Texas University has a fairly comprehensive evaluation process in place. Kentucky, which started later than many programs, has integrated an evaluation into its program. Issues include not only whether or not students remain at the agency once they complete their required pay back time, but also how effective Title IV-E program graduates are in their work with clients. The latter is much more difficult to demonstrate, but will be necessary if we want to provide support for Title IV-E funding.

Respondents also mentioned the need for more information about implementing Title IV-E programs. Because respondents to Zlotnik's survey expressed the same concern (Zlotnik & Cornelius, 2000), it appears that more programs are learning about Title IV-E, but don't know how to implement it. BSW program directors located in states where the public child welfare agency either does not hire BSWs or is not convinced that Title IV-E is the best way to train child welfare workers are often frustrated when they hear success stories from other states. And the exclusion of funding for private social work programs unless they can come up with a cash match or work with a public university has limited the availability of training, even though it can be argued that public universities are more cost-efficient.

While not all schools are interested in Title IV-E funding, interested schools should have ready access to information about funding availability and application procedures. It is difficult to do this on a national level because each state has developed its own way of administering Title IV-E funds. However, state and regional social work consortia should be able to help disseminate some of this information.

Finally, the information in this report should be interpreted in context. One of the limitations of the data is that program directors may have interpreted the questions differently than they were intended. Respondents were unclear about two questions, one on allowing students from other states to participate in the program and one on how soon after receiving their BSW graduates could enter an MSW program. Because the number of BSW programs receiving Title IV-E funding constantly changes, we were unable to determine how many programs receiving Title IV-E educational funds did not respond to the survey.

Finally, individual schools reported the information. This may give more weight to states where a number of schools reported and skew the information on stipends and tuition. But, because different programs within states reported receiving different amounts for stipends and tuition, each program within a state was included in the analysis.

CONCLUSION

A relatively small number of BSW programs are working with state child welfare agencies to provide Title IV-E stipends and educational programs that support students who are willing to commit to working in public child welfare after graduation. These programs have been developed based on prior research that shows child welfare workers with a social work degree usually are more effective than those who have other kinds of degrees (Albers et al., 1993; Dhooper et al., 1990) and that workers with social work backgrounds have lower turnover rates (Russell, 1987; Vinokur-Kaplan, 1991).

Although Title IV-E funding is available to BSW programs in only about half of the states, in the states where it is available, a number of workers have received much of their pre-service training while in practicum and through child welfare courses. States are able to waive much of the pre-service training for these new workers who are able to quickly move into communities, understand family problems and take on more complicated cases. This has allowed newly hired Title IV-E graduates to be ahead of the curve when they begin work in child welfare agencies.

REFERENCES

Albers, E.C., Reilly, T., & Rittner, B. (1993). Children in foster care: Possible factors affecting permanency planning. *Child and Adolescent Social Work Journal, 10*, 329-341.

Costin, L., Karger, J., & Stoesz, D. (1996). *The politics of child abuse in America.* New York: Oxford University Press.

Dhooper, S.S., Royse, D.D., & Wolfe, L.C. (1990). Does social work make a difference? *Social Work Education, 35*, 57-61.

Hilbert, J. (2001). Violence in the family: A story in need of an ending. In A. Sallee, H. Lawson & K. Briar-Lawson (Eds.) *Innovative practices with vulnerable children and families.* (pp. 105-120). Dubuque, Iowa: Eddie Bowers Publishing, Inc.

Lieberman, A.A., Hornby, H., & Russell, M. (1988). Analyzing the educational backgrounds and work experiences of child welfare personnel: A national study. *Social Work, 33*, 485-489.

Olsen, L. & Holmes, W.H. (1982). Educating child welfare workers: The effect of professional training on service delivery. *Journal of Education for Social Work, 18,* 94-102.

Pecora, P., Briar, K., & Zlotnik, J. (1989). *Addressing the program and personnel crisis in child welfare: A social work response.* Silver Spring, MD: National Association of Social Workers.

Russell, M. (1987). *1987 national study of public child welfare job requirements.* Portland, ME: University of Southern Maine, National Child Welfare Resource Center for Management and Administration.

Smith, B. (2001). Child welfare and substance abuse: Toward partnerships with parents and communities. In A. Sallee, H. Lawson & K. Briar-Lawson (Eds.) *Innovative practices with vulnerable children and families.* (pp. 105-120). Dubuque, Iowa: Eddie Bowers Publishing, Inc.

Vinokur-Kaplan, D. (1991). Job satisfaction among social workers in public and voluntary child welfare agencies. *Child Welfare, 70,* 81-91.

Zlotnik, J. (1997). *Preparing the workforce for family-centered practice: Social work education and public human services partnerships.* Alexandria, VA: Council on Social Work Education.

Zlotnik, J. (1998). *Historical analysis of the implementation of federal policy: A case study of accessing Title IV-E funds to support social work education.* Unpublished doctoral dissertation, University of Maryland, College Park.

Zlotnik, J. & Cornelius, L. (2000). Preparing social work students for child welfare careers: The use of Title IV-E training funds in social work education. *Journal of Baccalaureate Social Work Education, 5,* 1-14.

Do Collaborations
with Schools of Social Work
Make a Difference
for the Field of Child Welfare?
Practice, Retention and Curriculum

Maria Scannapieco
Kelli Connell-Corrick

SUMMARY. Historically, the profession of social work has held a leadership role in the field of child welfare. Opportunities provided in a number of significant public policies allow schools of social work to be eligible to receive Title IV-E funding for professional development of child welfare workers. Today, hundreds of these partnerships throughout the country (Zlotnik, 1997) are spending millions of federal dollars to professionally educate Bachelor of Social Work and Master of Social Work students for careers in child welfare. Unfortunately, there is not a corresponding proliferation of evaluation research to measure the effectiveness of these partnerships. This article provides a comprehensive description and evaluation of a partnership

---

Maria Scannapieco, PhD, is Professor and Director, University of Texas, Arlington, School of Social Work, Center for Child Welfare, Box 19129, Arlington, TX 76019-0129 (E-mail: mscannapieco@uta.edu).

Kelli Connell-Corrick, LMSW, is Assistant Professor, University of Texas El Paso.

[Haworth co-indexing entry note]: "Do Collaborations with Schools of Social Work Make a Difference for the Field of Child Welfare? Practice, Retention and Curriculum." Scannapieco, Maria and Kelli Connell-Corrick. Co-published simultaneously in *Journal of Human Behavior in the Social Environment* (The Haworth Social Work Practice Press, an imprint of The Haworth Press, Inc.) Vol. 7, No. 1/2, 2003, pp. 35-51; and: *Charting the Impacts of University-Child Welfare Collaboration* (ed: Katharine Briar-Lawson, and Joan Levy Zlotnik) The Haworth Social Work Practice Press, an imprint of The Haworth Press, Inc., 2003, pp. 35-51. Single or multiple copies of this article are available for a fee from The Haworth Document Delivery Service [1-800-HAWORTH, 9:00 a.m. - 5:00 p.m. (EST). E-mail address: getinfo@haworthpressinc.com].

between a school of social work and a state department of child protective services. *[Article copies available for a fee from The Haworth Document Delivery Service: 1-800-HAWORTH. E-mail address: <getinfo@haworthpressinc.com> Website: <http://www.HaworthPress.com> © 2003 by The Haworth Press, Inc. All rights reserved.]*

KEYWORDS. MSW, child welfare, evaluation, partnership

Since the early 1900s, there has been an evolution in child welfare and its connection to schools of social work in the United States. Zlotnik (1997a) outlines a 60-year history of collaborations between schools of social work and child welfare agencies that led to today's proliferation of partnerships between schools of social work and state child welfare agencies. Most notably child welfare's loss of status among social workers in the 1980s resulted in a special meeting of the National Association of Social Workers (NASW) in 1986 to address the issue (Kadushin & Martin, 1988). Since then, schools of social work have collaborated with public child welfare agencies to improve child welfare standing in the profession.

Opportunities provided in a number of significant public policies (Child Welfare Provisions of the Social Security Act, 1935; Public Law 96-272), allows schools of social work to be eligible to receive Title IV-E funding for professional development of child welfare workers. Schools of social work in collaboration with state child welfare agencies can be funded through Title IV-E for curriculum development, classroom instruction, and field instruction that are related to the mission of the child welfare agency. Today hundreds of these partnerships throughout the country (Zlotnik, 1997b) are spending millions of federal dollars to professionally educate Bachelor of Social Work and Master of Social Work students for careers in child welfare. Unfortunately, there is not a corresponding proliferation of evaluation research that attempts to measure the effectiveness of these partnerships. The federal government, however, is becoming increasingly interested in outcomes, and in some states are initiating reporting systems.

Through the collaborative efforts between The University of Texas at Arlington (UTA) and the Texas Department of Protective and Regulatory Services (TDPRS), evaluation objectives have been identified and measured. This article describes three areas of evaluation, which focus on both the school and agency: The impact on child welfare practice in the agency, the retention of child welfare workers, and curriculum development.

Review of the Literature

The objective of this literature review is twofold: identifying the extant research describing the impact of social work education on child welfare and retention of employees in child welfare. The empirical literature addressing the impact of reintroducing the profession of social work to the child welfare field and retention is sparse. Sixteen articles that relate to the impact of social work education on child welfare and the retention of child welfare employees were identified (Albers, Reilly & Rittner, 1993; Booz-Allen & Hamilton, 1987; Burmham, 1997; Cicero-Reese and Black, 1998; Dhooper, Royse & Wolfe, 1990; Jones, 1966; Lieberman, Hornby & Russell, 1988; Markeiwicz, 1996; Moran, Frans & Gibson, 1995; Olsen & Holmes, 1982; Reagh, 1994; Rycraft, 1990; Rycraft 1994; Samantrai, 1994; Vinokur-Kaplan, 1987; Vinokur-Kaplan, 1991). Other research found focuses on the development, identification and evaluation of necessary competencies in traineeship programs (Cahn, 1997; Hodges, Morgan and Johnston, 1993); and the differences in field practice between BSW and MSW education child welfare workers (Alperin, 1996).

In assessing the impact of social work education to child welfare and in examining the research on retention, many different variables were studied throughout the literature. This review will only include the studies that prove to be most relevant to the concepts in this study. Five general areas were identified: job performance and preparedness, service delivery, retention, impact of a social work degree and social work values. The most applicable and significant finding will be presented.

Job Performance and Preparedness. Supervisors rated MSWs as performing the highest in terms of overall performance as compared to all non-MSW degreed staff when training and years of experience were controlled (Booz-Allen and Hamilton, 1987). The MSW degree was also rated as producing the best-prepared employee for the job and requiring the least amount of supervision and training when given a hypothetical new employee applicant (Booz-Allen and Hamilton, 1987). MSWs also rated themselves as being best prepared for and most knowledgeable about child welfare work (Lieberman, Hornby & Russell, 1988).

Service Delivery. MSWs were found to be more effective in delivering substitute services; BSWs were most capable of providing supportive services to children (i.e., day mental health treatment). Overall social work trained staff were better than non-social work trained staff at delivering the majority of services to families and children (Olsen and Holmes, 1982). Social work trained staff were more effective than other staff in providing substitute care and supportive services, environmental services and planning for ongoing contact between biological families and children in foster care (Olsen and Holmes, 1992). In looking at effectiveness in permanency planning, social work trained child welfare workers were more likely to have a permanent plan for a child in foster care within three years when compared to workers with other degrees (Albers, Reilly and Rittner, 1993).

Retention. Two qualitative studies reviewed looked specifically at why caseworkers in public child welfare choose to stay with the agency (Reagh, 1994; Rycraft, 1994) and one qualitative study looked at why MSW caseworkers leave a public child welfare agency (Samantrai, 1992). Rycraft (1994) found four factors that influence retention, including the caseworker's mission and commitment to helping others, especially children; the goodness of fit between the individual and the job assignment; supervision that is adequate and available for guidance; and the worker's professional and personal investment in public child welfare. Other studies have found that the intrinsic rewards of public child welfare practice, personal accomplishment in helping others and the intertwining of personal and professional sense of identify additionally contribute to the reasons why workers remain employed in child welfare while others leave (Reagh, 1994). On the other hand, reasons for MSW educated workers termination include burnout, when no other alternative for transferring within the agency is available, and relationship with immediate supervisor (Samantrai, 1992). It is interesting to note that when supervision is viewed favorably it is cited as a reason for remaining in child welfare (Rycraft, 1994), while when viewed unfavorably it is a reason for terminating employment (Samantrai, 1992). Importantly, in all of the studies reviewed, a preference for working with vulnerable children and families was an emergent theme regardless of the additional stressors that may affect a decision to leave (Reagh, 1994; Rycraft, 1994; Samantrai, 1992).

Impact of social work degree. In an evaluation of the partnership in Florida between a child welfare agency and university, most of the Title IV-E stipend graduates responded that the skills acquired in their MSW program were effectively used; two-thirds felt that they were able to efficiently change the agency; and all of the respondents reported personal changes, such as knowledge acquisition, ethics awareness, coping skills, and assertiveness (Burmham, 1997). Administrators reported that the child welfare agency benefited from the partnership, and saw the MSW program employees as advocates for family preservation and family-based services (Burmham, 1997).

Social Work Values. In assessing impact of a social work degree on the management of a human service agency with respect to values and worker attitude, MSW students scored higher on the issues of social justice, individual freedom, human nature and collective identity than MBA students (Moran, Frans and Gibson, 1995). MSWs were also more effective managers in human service organizations since they tended to hold values and possess personal qualities important to the job when age, gender, study design and undergraduate education were controlled (Moran, Frans and Gibson, 1995). MSWs had the highest mean scores on a social work values instrument when compared to BSWs, who ranked second, followed by BA/BSs and MA/MSs (Dhooper, Royse and Wolfe, 1990). Although these findings are substantively significant, the results did not reach statistical significance.

As evidenced by the lack of research examining the impact of social work education on the professionalism of child welfare and the need for more studies examining the dynamics involved in retaining social work educated employees, empirical studies are greatly needed. The three empirical studies presented in this paper that are part of an overall evaluation add to the current body of research in this area. The first study describes the impact of an MSW on a child welfare agency; the second study describes findings from a survey that assessed the retention of child welfare employees who participated in a Title IV-E program; and the third study describes the infusion of child welfare content into the Master's curriculum at a university. Providing a detailed description of all results of the three studies is beyond the scope of this article. Therefore, only the most relevant and significant results will be presented.

Description of the Title IV-E Partnership

The University of Texas at Arlington (UTA) School of Social Work through the Center for Child Welfare entered into a partnership agreement with the Texas Department of Protective and Regulatory Services, Child Protective Services Division (CPS), Region 03 (Dallas–Fort Worth Area) in September 1994. This partnership was based on a Title IV-E contract to provide professional education towards the Master of Social Work Degree for current employees of the agency and the recruitment of BSW and MSW students into the field of child welfare.

The majority, 179, of students who have participated in this program have done so as a full-time CPS employee. Additionally, 133 BSW and MSW students have been recruited into the field of child welfare through this program. All students who choose to enter the program are required to focus their studies on family and children content areas (UTA does not have fields of specialization) and to do one field placement with CPS. See Scannapieco, Bolen and Connell (2000) for a detailed discussion of the Title IV-E program.

Partnership Arrangement

UTA and the Texas Department of Protective and Regulatory Services take pride in the collaborative nature of the partnership. Since the inception of the Title IV-E contract there has been a joint committee made up of CPS employees and School of Social Work faculty. The committee serves an advisory function for curriculum development and evaluation.

Evaluation and planning have also been integral tasks of the committee. To guide the efforts of the committee, goals and operationalized objectives were established and appropriate methods for analyzing each objective were specified. Efforts to analyze these objectives are three-fold, and provide the rationale for the three studies described in this paper. The first was to determine the impact and success of the Title IV-E program from both the students' and the larger community's perspective (Scannapieco, Bolen & Connell, 2000). The second was to determine the retention of IV-E participants in the agency (Scannapieco, Faulkner & Connell, 1999a). The third, an on-going effort, was to determine the current level of child welfare content in courses so that it could be used as a baseline for annual analyses (Scannapieco, Faulkner, & Connell, 1999b; Scannapieco & Bolen, 1998).

STUDY 1: PERCEIVED IMPACT OF IV-E PROGRAM

The main objective of this evaluation was to determine the impact and success of the MSW Title IV-E program from both the students' and the larger community's perspective. This section presents the findings of surveys administered to both MSW Title IV-E students and to supervisors and administrators of Texas Department of Protective and Regulatory Services (TDPRS). In both surveys, respondents were asked demographic information as well as information about their status at work/in school. Students were also asked a series of questions concerning their perception of the impact of their Masters education on their professional aptitude. Supervisors/administrators were asked their perception of whether employees with MSWs could be differentiated from Bachelor-level employees.

Methodology

The student survey was mailed to all current or past MSW Title IV-E students enrolled at UTA and currently employed at Child Protective Services. Of the 118 surveys mailed, 50 were returned, for a response rate of 42%. The administrative survey was mailed to all supervisors and higher-level administrators in TDPRS. Of the 103 surveys mailed, 46 were returned, for a response rate of 45%. Both of the surveys captured basic demographic information, followed by a series of questions assessing the perceived impact of the Title IV-E program on CPS as an agency, students participating in the IV-E program, including both professional and personal implications, and whether service delivery to CPS clients has been changed due to the IV-E program.

Student Survey Results

The mean age of the student survey was 34.6; eighty six (86)% of the student respondents were female. The questions were divided into four categories: Relationship of Employee to TDPRS, Relationship of Employee to Community, Employee and Social Work profession and Employee and Skill Acquisition. Approximately 50% of the students agreed or strongly agreed that their Masters education had improved their skills and relationship with TDPRS and the profession. Minority students were more likely to report that their education had improved their relationship with TDPRS ($p < .10$). Seventy percent (70%) of the students report that they have a better ability to use various interventions with clients, and 74% reported having more advanced assessment skills. Approximately 50% of students agreed that their education had improved not only their relationship with their employers, community and the profession, but also positively affected their acquisition of skills.

Administrators Survey Results

The mean age of the administrators survey was 44.5. Eighty percent (80%) of the administrators' respondents were female. Most of the respondents (80%) were supervisors, while nineteen percent (19%) of the respondents were administrators. The questions were divided into five areas: Relationship of Employee to TDPRS, Approach to Work, Relationship of Employee to Community, Employee and Social Work Profession and Employee and Skill Acquisition. The overall perception of Title IV-E program was always either positive or neutral; no negative scores were offered. Forty seven percent (47%) agreed that MSW's have a better ability to use various interventions with clients than do Bachelor-level employees. Respondents stated that MSW's have a better understanding of social work values and ethics (45.5% and 50% respectively). The highest response was that MSW's have a much higher level of commitment to TDPRS than do Bachelor's level employee. Administrators with either a Masters degree or a major in social work consistently rated their Masters-level workers as better than Bachelor's level employees.

Comparison of Students' to Administrators' Perception of Impact

Students consistently rated the impact of the Masters education as more beneficial than did administrators. Administrators exceeded students' perception on four questions and rated MSW's as having more commitment to TDPRS, a better knowledge of community resources, more creativity in job, and better communication skills with clients. The combination of the Masters degree and the social work degree made the most difference in perception.

STUDY 2:
FOLLOW-UP OF TITLE IV-E GRADUATES: TRACKING CHILD WELFARE RETENTION

Another goal of the collaboration is to improve retention of IV-E participants in the field of child welfare. Scannapieco, Faulkner and Connell (1999a) conducted a survey of stipend participants who successfully graduated with a degree in social work. Since 1995, 128 total stipend participants had graduated. The purpose of this survey was to examine the characteristics of graduates, especially related to their choice of employment and whether they felt there had been an increase in social work professionalism since the influx of social workers at CPS.

Two survey instruments were developed and participants received both. One was designed for students who had graduated and were still employed by CPS, the other was developed for students who graduated and had eventually left the agency's employment.

Results for Entire Cohort

Of the 128 surveys mailed, 83 total graduates responded for a 64% response rate. Significantly more females than males responded and significantly more whites than non-whites responded. The findings for the combined surveys were significant in two areas, salary and increased professionalism. Graduates who left CPS report a statistically significant increase in salary even while controlling for race and gender. Graduates who remain at the agency full-time report an average monthly income of $355.00 while those graduates who left CPS but still working full-time report a monthly income of $460.00, a difference of $105.00 per month ($p < .001$). When asked about increased professionalism, CPS workers stayed employed at the agency regardless of whether they felt there was an increase in professionalism because of their commitment to child welfare work, a finding also supported by previous research (Reagh, 1994; Rycraft, 1994). As interesting, the majority of workers (55%) who both stayed and left reported that there was an increase in professionalism.

Graduates Currently Employed at CPS

Of the 58 total respondents, the majority was women and Caucasian. Investigation and generic units employed nearly half (44%) of 58 respondents.

Eighty one percent (81%) of the respondents were CPS workers. This is particularly important when looking at the mean employment experience of 5 years. Therefore, workers are remaining in positions that give them direct access to children in families where abuse or neglect is suspected.

Of the 58 respondents, 69% felt there was an increase in professionalism on the job since the influx of BSW and MSW social workers to the agency. Seventy-nine percent (79%) of the 53 respondents reported they were likely or very likely to be employed at CPS in the year 2000. When asked where they were likely to seek employment if they were to leave CPS, 50% reported that they would continue to work in the area of children and families.

The most frequent reason to remain employed at CPS was a commitment to the work (77.6%), as also evidenced by previous research (Reach, 1994; Rycraft, 1994); and the second most cited reason is flexible schedule (74.1%). Finally, when asked whether they felt there was an increase in professionalism since the influx of BSW and MSW social workers, 69% felt there was an increase.

Graduates Who Left CPS

Twenty-five (25) surveys were returned from graduates who were no longer employed by CPS. Of the 25 total respondents, the majority was female and Caucasian. Forty percent (40%) of the 25 respondents reported currently working in the area of families and children. Other respondents were working in related areas such as school social work and juvenile justice.

Salary was reported as the most frequent reason for leaving CPS at 76%. Dissatisfaction with workload, supervision, and promotion were additional reasons. Eighty-eight percent (81%) of the respondents reported an increase in salary after leaving CPS with an average monthly salary of $2,737.98, a $105.00 monthly difference (p < .001).

Of those who left 40% of the respondents felt there was an increase in professionalism since the influx of BSW and MSW social workers. However, it is important to consider that the average total length of CPS employment was only 3 years with a range between 3 months to 11 years. It is possible that many graduates who had prior experience as well as new CPS employees changed jobs shortly after graduation and were not available to see the positive change that current employees report.

STUDY 3: ANNUAL SURVEY OF CHILD WELFARE CONTENT

One of the overall goals of the Title IV-E program is to infuse child welfare content into the MSW curriculum, both on the foundation and advanced level.

The Advisory committee has been instrumental in the direction that curriculum development has taken. Faculty have been receptive to content needs expressed by CPS staff and have contributed to syllabus, course and module development. Table 1 includes the curriculum modules have been developed to date.

These modules are available to all faculty and instructors in order to facilitate the infusion of child welfare content into the social work curriculum, as well as schools of social work nationwide and CPS staff and administrators. This ensures that, as teaching assignments change, content will not be dependent upon specific faculty members. In addition to the modules, Table 2 details syllabi and courses that have been developed through this contract specific to child welfare.

In sum, the development and utilization of these curriculum modules and syllabi ensure that child welfare content can be infused into the foundation and advanced social work curriculum. Part of the scope of the Title IV-E project is to improve child welfare content in MSW courses already being offered and to make recommendations for future courses. These courses not only benefit the Title IV-E students, but also make all students more cognizant of the critical issues of child welfare.

Methodology

All University MSSW instructors were notified of the survey and were asked to allow a Center representative to administer the survey in their class.

TABLE 1. UTA Child Welfare Modules

Title	Date Developed
Research and Evaluation: Child Welfare Course Pack	1997
Issues in Child Welfare: An International Perspective	1998
Direct Practice I: Child Welfare Infusion	1998
Substance Abuse: Materials for Classroom Instruction	1998
Lesbian, Gay, Bisexual and Transgender Youths	1998
Child Welfare Policy	1998
Administrative and Community Practice in Child Welfare Settings and Context	1999
Substance Abuse and Child Maltreatment	1999
Family Therapy and Child Welfare	1999
Working with Parents and Children with Disabilities	1999
Working with Fathers and Boys	2000
Direct Practice and Child Welfare II: Theoretical Frameworks	2000

TABLE 2 UTA Child Welfare Courses

Title	Date Developed
Advanced Administration for Children and Families	1997
Child and Youth Policy	1998
Child Maltreatment and Substance Abuse	1999
Brief Therapy for a Managed Care Environment	1999

Center representatives attended each class after obtaining permission from the Instructor. Before the respondents completed the survey, the definition for child welfare, deriving from the Encyclopedia of Social Work (Liederman, 1995), was read to the students. All students taking the survey were instructed to complete it only once. The questionnaire was brief, having been designed to be completed in less than 5 minutes.

RESULTS

The final sample size was 317, a response rate of 69%. The surveyed students were representative of the larger population of students on gender, ethnicity, and their Title IV-E status.

Demographics and Related Questions

Distributions were uniformly skewed towards females, non-Title IV-E students, Direct Practice concentrations, and Caucasians, reflecting the overrepresentation of these students in the Masters program. Sixty-two (62%) of the respondents entered the program within the past years and 61% were enrolled full-time. Forty-three percent (43%) of the surveyed students stated that it was "possible" that they would enter into child welfare following graduation. Thirty-four percent (34%) stated that they were either "likely" or "very likely" to work in child welfare upon graduation. Only 22% reported that there was no likelihood in working in child welfare upon graduation. Sixty percent (60%) of respondents stated that they thought that an adequate emphasis was currently being placed on child welfare content, and 49% of respondents felt that there should be more emphasis on child welfare content in the future.

Courses

The following section outlines the five content areas of social work (human behavior, policy, administration and community practice, research and direct practice) and required foundation courses. The results of the survey for each social work content area will be presented in Table 3. All courses were scored on a Likert scale from 1 ("Very Little") to 4 ("A Great Deal"), with a score of 2.5 representing a neutral position. For a comparison between the baseline and current study, please see Scannapieco, Faulkner & Connell (1999b).

Table 3 describes the results of the survey, and the perception of child welfare content in the MSW curriculum. Of all the courses, foundation and required courses had the greatest number of responses overall, most likely because the majority of these courses were taken in the first year.

For the advanced courses, the highest rated social work content area was policy. Mean scores ranged from 1.33 to 3.91, with more courses scored at 2.5 or greater. With all courses included, 51% of students rated these courses as having "some" or "a great deal" of child welfare content; with Issues in Child Welfare eliminated, 47% of students rated them as such.

Overall, ACP courses, excluding the Management of Children's Agencies and Programs course in which the mean score was 3.36, were uniformly rated low on child welfare content, with the mean ranging from 1.0 to 2.22. For the Human behavior content area, five courses were rated at 2.5 or better, and 44% of the respondents rated human behavior courses as "some" or "a great deal." Similar to the human behavior findings, 45% of students rated Direct Practice courses as having "some" or "a great deal" of child welfare content. While 80% of the students rated courses *with* a child/family focus as having "some" or "a great deal" of child welfare content, only 29% of the students rated Direct Practice courses *without* a child/family focus at these levels.

TABLE 3. Foundation and Advanced Courses

Area of Social Work Course	% Rated as Having "Some" or "a Great Deal" of Child Welfare Content	Range of Mean Scores
Foundation and Required	28%	1.21-2.63
Advanced Courses		
Policy	51%	1.33-3.91
Administrative and Community Practice	28%	1.00-3.36
Human Behavior	44%	1.27-3.48
Direct Practice	45%	1.33-3.77
Total for Advanced Courses	41%	

When foundation courses were compared to advanced courses, advanced courses were somewhat superior in offering child welfare content. One possible reason for this is that by the advanced year, students are more attuned to child welfare issues or have a more global view of child welfare practice. In addition to child welfare content in courses, the following section further describes additional demographic attributes of MSW students and other bivariate comparisons.

Other Comparisons

Students who stated a desire to work in child welfare after graduation were also more likely to state child welfare as their specialization and to have more years of both professional and volunteer experience in child welfare. Minorities, students specializing in child welfare, and those entering more recently were more likely to endorse a greater need for child welfare content in the future. Minorities were more likely than Caucasians to report a need for more emphasis on child welfare content in the future. Because this finding was found in the baseline and 1999 surveys, this finding is substantively important. Additionally, Minorities were likely to have an ACP concentration, to be Title IV-E students, to have more years of professional experience, and to endorse that salary was more of an issue upon graduation. A possible explanation for these findings is that, of the minority respondents in this survey, more minorities are choosing the field of child welfare, have a greater interest in child welfare and are Title IV-E students.

In conclusion, a substantively noteworthy difference exists for minorities and non-minorities as well and interesting salary perceptions of child welfare. Although assessing the underlying reasons for these differences is beyond the scope of this study, they should be explored in the future.

DISCUSSION

Perceived impact on child welfare practice. The purpose of both the student and administrator surveys was to determine the perceived impact of the Title IV-E program on child welfare practice. More specifically, we wish to assess whether having a MSW positively influences the quality of child welfare practice. Although the sample size was small it was representative of all employees who receive a stipend to obtain an MSW and of all administrators at CPS. Determining the impact of educational level on the quality of practice is a difficult task and one that the field is struggling with currently. The use of social worker and administrator perceptions as a measure of impact on practice is limited and subjective, but is used throughout the empirical literature (Burmham, 1997).

Concerning the student survey, it is encouraging to note that approximately 50% of students agreed that their education had improved not only their relationships with their employers, community, and the profession, but also had positively affected their acquisition of skills. The findings were not as encouraging for administrators. Thirty percent to 45% of administrators agreed that MSWs exhibited better professional relationships, skills, and employment dynamics than Bachelors level workers. On the other hand, 22% to 29% disagreed that workers with MSWs were better than Bachelors level workers, suggesting that administrators were mixed in their perception of the impact of workers with MSWs.

Another aim was to determine whether specific factors were correlated with students' and administrators' perceptions of the Title IV-E program's impact. For administrators, the most important factor appeared to be the administrator's level of education. Administrators with either a Masters degree, as compared to a Bachelors degree, or with a major in social work, as compared to another major, consistently rated Masters level workers as better than Bachelors level workers. MSWs consistently had the highest scores, with administrators; Bachelors in something other than social work or psychology had the lowest scores. Administrators with BSWs, a Bachelors degree in psychology, or a Masters degree in something other than social work had similar scores, although BSWs had marginally higher scores than the other two groups.

These findings indicate that it is the combination of the social work degree and the Masters level education that made the most difference in perception. Historically, child welfare, more so than other areas, is inimitably identified with social work values and ethics. Administrators are probably more able to recognize the advantage of having an MSW in the provision of services. In this perspective, MSWs are both better at delivering and recognizing child welfare services that are steeped in social work values and ethics. This perspective is based, however, upon the assumption that the delivery of services based upon social work values and ethics are superior to another model. Moreover, this issue cannot be resolved within this article and may be more philosophical than empirical.

This study indicates that those individuals with the most training in recognizing the proper application of a social work model believe that MSWs are better able than Bachelors level workers to apply this model across domains. From this perspective, the Title IV-E program is effective in developing skills, values, and ethics in students that are pertinent and critical to the appropriate delivery of services. In sum, the impact study evaluates the identified goals of the Title IV-E project in a substantive manner.

Retention study. The responses from each survey individually and combined yielded some interested findings. Although income was cited as the most frequent reason for leaving employment with CPS, the state of Texas, unrelated to the findings of this study, changed its pay plan and gave all CPS staff salary increases. This pay increase occurred after the completion of this survey, so the reasons for leaving might be different now that CPS salaries are more competitive. Another reason cited for leaving the agency was supervision, which is consistent with earlier findings (Samantrai, 1994). In this study and in previous studies the commitment to the work is cited as one reason for staying employed in child welfare (Reagh, 1994; Rycraft, 1994; Samantrai, 1988). More importantly, most 70% of those still employed at CPS feel that a social work degree has affected the increase in professionalism in the agency, a finding mirrored in the previous study in this article.

Curriculum study. Since the inception of the Title IV-E program, the infusion of child welfare material into the classroom has been of great importance. Although it is too early to adequately discuss the effects of this infusion, the dissemination of child welfare content in classes affects not only IV-E students, but also the entire MSSW population at this university. Through the development of modules and courses, knowledge of and the difficult issues surrounding child welfare are brought to the attention of all students, with the purposeful hope of drawing more students into child welfare and educating those already involved.

CONCLUSIONS

Since the inception of the social work profession in the late nineteenth century and through the efforts of individuals like Jane Addams' of the settlement house movement and Mary Richmond of the charity organization movement, the social work profession recognized the responsibility to address the social problems related to child welfare (Addams, 1903, as cited in Pumphrey & Pumphrey, 1961, p. 279; Richmond, 1897, as cited in Pumphrey & Pumphrey, 1961, 289). "The authority and permission for social workers to act in relation to these problems has been sanctioned by the community, the client group served, and the profession" (Kadushin & Martin, 1988, p. 5). The challenges child welfare professionals face in the new millennium are even greater than those faced by Jane Addams and her colleagues: crack/cocaine epidemic, domestic violence, HIV/AIDS, identification and reporting of maltreatment, twofold increase in population. Child maltreatment continues to rise, out of home placements are increasing and the underlying correlates of this social problems are more and more complex. Families that enter the child welfare system are from the global community and present challenges and opportunities for the field. The social work field must respond by understanding client's culture and values, and it demands professionals who have critical thinking capacity.

Schools of Social Work and public child welfare agencies that collaborate to access Title IV-E funding are presented with many opportunities to meet the needs of the ever changing child welfare system. The overall effect of bringing the social work profession back to child welfare is difficult to measure but as demonstrated through this article, there are great benefits for the school, the agency, and most importantly the families and children that are the focus of professional development are great. Title IV-E funding is essential to the specialized training and education need for child welfare workers to address the most serious of our society's ills, child maltreatment.

REFERENCES

Albers, E., Reilly, T. and Rittner, B. (1993). Children in foster care: Possible factors affecting permanency planning. *Child and Adolescent Social Work, 10*(4), 329-341.

Alperin, D. (1996) Graduate and undergraduate field placements in child welfare: Is there a difference? *The Journal of Baccalaureate Social Work, 2*(1), 109-124.

Booz-Allen and Hamilton, Inc. (1987). *The Maryland social work services job analysis and personnel qualifications study.* Prepared for The Department of Human Resources, State of Maryland, Baltimore, MD.

Burmham, M (1997, January). FIU evaluates its Title IV-E partnership. *Partnerships for Child Welfare, 5*(3), 3.

Cahn, K. (1997). Evaluating the impact of creative partnerships. *Partnerships for Child Welfare, 5* (4), 2, 12.

Cicero-Reese, B., and Black, P. (1998, February). Research suggests why child welfare workers stay on the job. *Partnerships for Child Welfare, 5*(5), 5-8.

Dhooper, S., Royse, D. and Wolfe, L. (1990). Does social work education make a difference? *Social Work, 35* (1), 57-61.

Hodges, V., Morgan, L. and Johnston, B. (1993). Educating for excellence in child welfare practice: A model for graduate training in intensive family preservation. *Journal of Teaching in Social Work, 7* (1), 31-49.

Jones, B. (1966). Non-professional workers in professional foster family agencies. *Child Welfare, 45,* 313-325.

Kadushin, A. & Martin, J. (1988). *Child welfare services, fourth edition.* New York: Macmillan Publishing Company.

Lieberman, A., Hornby, H. and Russell, M. (1988). Analyzing the educational background and work experiences of child welfare personnel: a national study. *Social Work, 33* (6), 485-489.

Liederman, David S. (1995). Child welfare overview. In *Encyclopedia of social work* (19th ed., Vol. 1, pp. 424-433). NY: National Association of Social Workers.

Markiewicz, A. (1996). Recruitment and retention of social work personnel within public child welfare: a case study of a Victorian department. *Australian Social Work, 49* (4), 11-17.

Moran, J., Frans, D., and Gibson, P. (1995) A comparison of beginning MSW and MBA students on their aptitudes for human service management. *Journal of Social Work Education, 31* (1), 95-105.

Olsen, L. and Holmes, W. (1982). Educating child welfare workers: The effects of professional training on service delivery. *Journal of Education for Social Work, 18* (1), 94-102.

Pumphrey P. & Pumphrey, M. (1961). *The heritage of American social work.* New York: Columbia University Press.

Reagh, R. (1994). Public child welfare professionals–those who stay. *Journal of Sociology and Social Welfare,* 21 (3), 69-78.

Rycraft, J. (1990). The survivors: *A qualitative study of the retention of public child welfare workers.* Unpublished doctoral dissertation, University of Illinois Urbana-Champaign.

Rycraft, J. (1994). The party isn't over: The agency role in the retention of public child welfare caseworkers. *Social Work 39*(1), 75-80.

Samantrai, K. (1992). Factors in the decision to leave: retaining social workers with MSWs in public child welfare. *Social Work, 37* (5), 454-458.

Scannapieco, M. & Bolen, R. (1998). *The University of Texas at Arlington School of Social Work baseline survey of child welfare content in the current MSSW courses.* Arlington. University of Texas at Arlington, Center for Child Welfare.

Scannapieco, M., Bolen, R. & Connell, K. (2000). The Impact of professional social work education in child welfare: Assessing practice knowledge and skills. *Professional Development: The International Journal of Continuing Education, 3* (1), 44-56.

Scannapieco, M., Faulkner, C. & Connell, K. (1999a). *Follow-up study of Title IV-E graduates: Tracking child welfare retention.* Arlington, TX: Center for Child Welfare, University of Texas at Arlington.

Scannapieco, M., Faulkner, C., & Connell, K. (1999b). *University of Texas at Arlington School of Social Work Annual Survey of Child Welfare Content in Current MSSW Courses.* Arlington, TX: Center for Child Welfare, University of Texas at Arlington.

Vinokur-Kaplan, D. (1987). Where did they go? A national follow-up of child welfare trainees. *Child Welfare, LXVI*(5), 411-421.

Vinokur-Kaplan, D. (1991). Job satisfaction among social workers in public and voluntary child welfare agencies. *Child Welfare, LXX*(1), 81-91.

Zlotnik, J. (1997a). Highlights of a 60-year history. *Partnerships for Child Welfare,* 5, 3, 6.

Zlotnik, J. (1997b). Results of CSWE Title IV-E Survey. *Partnerships for Child Welfare,* 5, 3-4.

Preparing Students
for Public Child Welfare:
Evaluation Issues and Strategies

Nancy Feyl Chavkin

J. Karen Brown

SUMMARY. Universities across the nation are attempting to increase the number of workers employed in child welfare, but thus far there has not been a systematic evaluation effort of these university/agency partnerships. This article addresses evaluation strategies and issues for preparing students for public child welfare by identifying eight beginning steps for university/agency partnerships to consider in developing an evaluation plan. Following the identification of the eight steps, the authors discuss key issues involved in evaluating university/agency child welfare partnerships and suggest recommendations for the future. *[Article copies available for a fee from The Haworth Document Delivery Service: 1-800-HAWORTH. E-mail address: <getinfo@haworthpressinc.com> Website: <http://www.HaworthPress.com> © 2003 by The Haworth Press, Inc. All rights reserved.]*

KEYWORDS. Evaluation, child welfare, training, partnerships, university, agency

---

Nancy Feyl Chavkin, PhD, and J. Karen Brown, PhD, are affiliated with Center for Children and Families, Department of Social Work, Southwest Texas State University, 601 University Drive, San Marcos, TX 78666.

[Haworth co-indexing entry note]: "Preparing Students for Public Child Welfare: Evaluation Issues and Strategies." Chavkin, Nancy Feyl, and J. Karen Brown. Co-published simultaneously in *Journal of Human Behavior in the Social Environment* (The Haworth Social Work Practice Press, an imprint of The Haworth Press, Inc.) Vol. 7, No. 1/2, 2003, pp. 53-66; and: *Charting the Impacts of University-Child Welfare Collaboration* (ed: Katharine Briar-Lawson, and Joan Levy Zlotnik) The Haworth Social Work Practice Press, an imprint of The Haworth Press, Inc., 2003, pp. 53-66. Single or multiple copies of this article are available for a fee from The Haworth Document Delivery Service [1-800-HAWORTH, 9:00 a.m. - 5:00 p.m. (EST). E-mail address: getinfo@haworthpressinc.com].

INTRODUCTION

The need for professionally prepared child welfare workers is indisputable. Leighninger and Ellett (1998) report that the work child welfare workers do is more challenging and with more difficult families than ever before in American history, but most of the employees entering the child welfare field do not have a professional social work education (Alperin, 1998; Baer & McLean, 1994). Lieberman, Hornby, and Russell (1988) found that only 28% of the nation's child welfare workers have a social work degree. Rome (1994) suggests that increasing student placements in child welfare will increase the number of social workers employed in child welfare. Zlotnik (1997) reports that with the aid of Title IV-B and Title IV-E funding, universities across the nation are attempting to increase the number of workers employed in child welfare, but thus far there has not been a systematic evaluation effort of these university/agency partnerships. This paper focuses on critical evaluation issues and strategies that are necessary if we want to prepare students effectively for public child welfare.

This paper addresses evaluation strategies and issues for preparing students for public child welfare by identifying eight beginning steps for university/agency partnerships to consider in developing an evaluation plan. Following the identification of the eight steps, the paper discusses key issues involved in evaluating university/agency child welfare partnerships and suggests recommendations for the future.

BEGINNING STEPS FOR EVALUATING UNIVERSITY/AGENCY PARTNERSHIPS

Knapp (1995) uses the term "thin" to describe the methodology literature to date about how to study partnerships, and his view is strongly supported by a search of the literature. Dryfoos (1994), working in the field of school-linked services, and Weiss and Greene (1992), working in the field of family support, were some of the first to argue that the traditional methodological approaches are not entirely appropriate for partnership evaluations.

University/agency partnerships that prepare students for public child welfare must be aware of the complexity of the issues involved and be open to developing their own individualized evaluation plans. Evaluators use many different frameworks for organizing evaluation plans, and there may be no one perfect plan for every university/agency partnership. Drawing on the work of leading evaluators, the authors have identified eight steps for evaluating university/agency partnerships. Although there are many helpful books on program evaluation (e.g. Gabor, Unrau, & Grinnell, 1998;) Jacobs, Williams, Kapuscik, & Kates, 1998; Rossi, Freeman & Lipsey, 1998; Royse & Thyer, 1996; and Weiss & Jacobs, 1988), no one book provides a clear recipe for how to handle the complexity of evaluating a university/agency partnership for preparing students for child welfare. Using these beginning steps (Table 1) as a guide, each partnership team should decide on its own individualized evaluation plan.

Step 1: Identify the Stakeholders

Identifying the stakeholders seems easy to most partnerships, but that is not always the case. When universities work with agencies, professors sometimes forget that the world is different outside of academia, and in turn, agencies find universities perplexing. The stakeholders have broadened beyond the typical professor and students. When a university joins with an agency, differing bureaucracies must be understood. Partnership teams must also make a decision early in the evaluation if the federal government, the state protective services agency, and/or the children/families who will be served by the project are the primary stakeholders. The evaluation plan must begin with all stakeholders identified and involved.

Weiss and Jacobs (1988) label step one as the needs assessment stage. It is the time when evaluators are establishing baseline information and reviewing existing data, identifying resources, unmet needs, and setting some broad goals. Others such as Melaville and Blank (1993) prefer to reframe the term to call it "taking stock." Whatever one calls this stage, the team needs to make sure that each of these stakeholders is involved from day one of the evaluation.

Step 2: Clarify the Goals

Although clarifying the goals of the university/agency partnership sounds simplistic, it really is one of the most difficult aspects of the partnership pro-

TABLE 1. Beginning Steps for Evaluating a Partnership

Beginning Steps for Evaluating a Partnership

1. Identify the Stakeholders
2. Clarify the Goals
3. Review Assumptions About Program Processes
4. Choose Indicators
5. Begin Collecting Information on Results
6. Analyze Information and Use It for Quality Improvement
7. Examine Outcomes
8. Assess Impact/Cost-Effectiveness

cess. It is amazing how many faculty and agency personnel cannot write a simple paragraph about what the goals of their projects are and what they expect to achieve if they accomplish the goals. If the stakeholders do write a simple paragraph about what they think the goals the partnership are, we often find that they have written markedly different goal statements. In one recent meeting of stakeholders, the agency partners saw the goal as to improve the lives of children and families in the child welfare system while the university partners saw the goal as increasing the number of social workers hired in the public child welfare system. These two goals, although not mutually exclusive, are different goals for the partnership. The partnership team needs all the stakeholders to participate in this step. This basic step is the foundation to a good evaluation.

Similarly, Hooper-Briar and Lawson (1994) discuss the necessity for a guiding vision in partnerships and collaboratives. They stress that the dialogue must begin with the children, youth, and family stakeholders and ask what outcomes they are expecting and then follow that with asking professional stakeholders about the benefits they expect to gain.

All of the indicators of success for the partnership should be built around the original goals that the partnership was designed to achieve. The partners then need to develop specific objectives to meet these goals. Assessment should focus on questions such as:

- Is the program in accord with its mission?
- What is it doing to reach its objectives?
- Is the program fulfilling the role mandated by the federal legislation?

Step 3: Review Assumptions about Program Processes

Once the partnership team is clear about the goals of the project, the team needs to draw a picture of what the assumptions about the program are. The partnership team needs to think about the assumptions the program is making, i.e., about what management structures and processes will work in their community. Many evaluators call this a logic model, a blue print, or graphic depiction because it shows the relationships between goals, outcomes, actions, and assumptions (see Figure 1 for an example from one university/agency). These linkages are very important to understanding what we know or think we know about our target population and the systems that serve them. Alter and Murty (1997) offer helpful insights about how to use logic modeling to evaluate practice. Freeman and Pennekamp (1988) call this step developing a shared theoretical map to improve practice.

FIGURE 1. LOGIC MODEL

GOAL: To Prepare Beginning Generalist Social Workers for Quality Practice in Child Welfare Settings

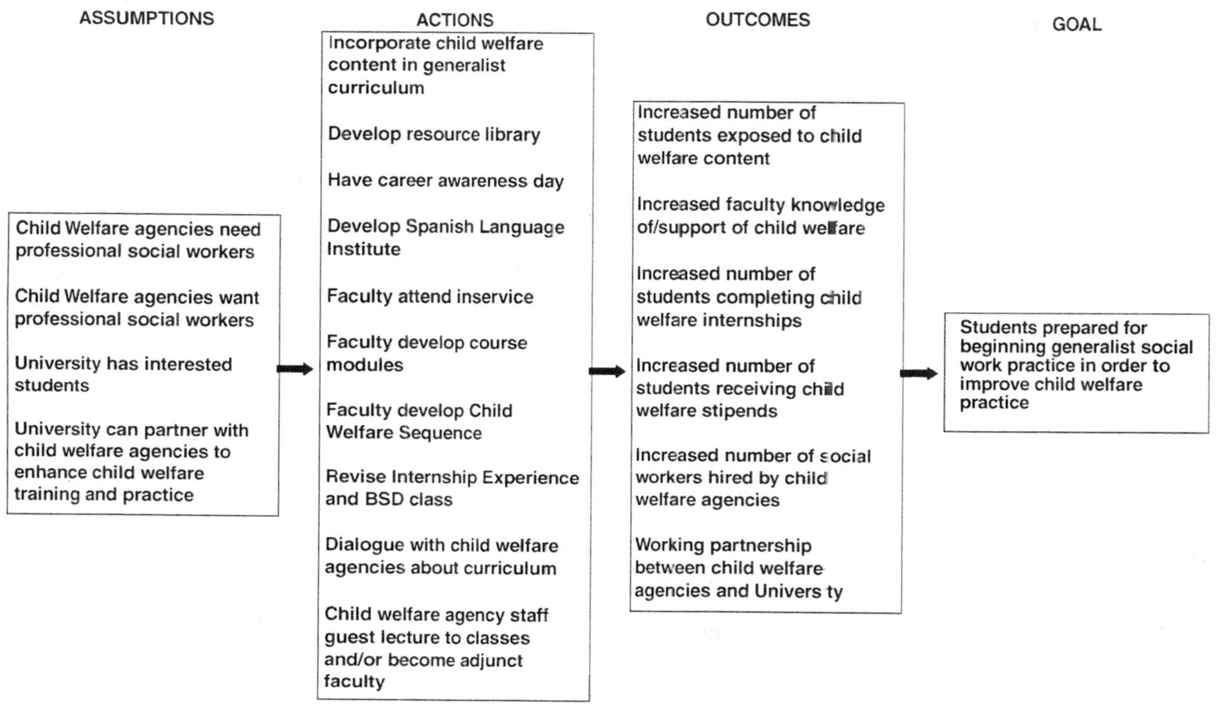

ASSUMPTIONS

- Child Welfare agencies need professional social workers
- Child Welfare agencies want professional social workers
- University has interested students
- University can partner with child welfare agencies to enhance child welfare training and practice

ACTIONS

- Incorporate child welfare content in generalist curriculum
- Develop resource library
- Have career awareness day
- Develop Spanish Language Institute
- Faculty attend inservice
- Faculty develop course modules
- Faculty develop Child Welfare Sequence
- Revise Internship Experience and BSD class
- Dialogue with child welfare agencies about curriculum
- Child welfare agency staff guest lecture to classes and/or become adjunct faculty

OUTCOMES

- Increased number of students exposed to child welfare content
- Increased faculty knowledge of/support of child welfare
- Increased number of students completing child welfare internships
- Increased number of students receiving child welfare stipends
- Increased number of social workers hired by child welfare agencies
- Working partnership between child welfare agencies and University

GOAL

Students prepared for beginning generalist social work practice in order to improve child welfare practice

Next the team needs to ask questions about the picture. Does information flow clearly? Is there a clear understanding of responsibilities and a system of accountability? These assumptions should drive program activities, and an evaluation will test the accuracy of the assumptions. If the results do not improve, either the assumptions were wrong or an anticipated event did not take place. The team needs to see if the program's activities are addressing the assumptions they made and if the outcomes they expect are being produced so that they can reach the goal. If this is not happening, the partnership team needs to reexamine the logic model.

Step 4: Choose Indicators

Indicators of success or outcomes should be established for all aspects of a program. Programs will want to assess whether they are achieving the goals they have set for meeting their students' needs by examining factors such as: numbers of students completing child welfare placements; student attitude, course taking, internship completion, internship performance, agency satisfaction, and impact on the community. Programmatic and management issues will need to be assessed by an appropriate set of indicators measuring the smoothness of operation, the flow of information, the system of accountability, and whether services are provided at the level of quality intended. Table 2 provides examples of indicators that many child welfare partnership programs are using.

Effective evaluations use several types of information to measure results. It is essential to establish short-term indicators of success to introduce the practice of continuous improvement in a program. Information on rates of attendance, instructor evaluations, and placement evaluations may provide a short-term means of assessing a program's progress towards its goals. Short-term indicators of program processes could include surveys of all levels of staff about their understanding of their responsibilities and their satisfaction with the system of accountability.

Step 5: Begin Collecting Information on Results

Strong evaluations collect information on participants, activities and services, staff and other resources, collaborative partners, and community perceptions. Sources of information may include: focus groups, community forums, surveys, registration or intake forms, staff activity logs, comparison groups that match similar groups, demographic data-

TABLE 2. Evaluation Indicators for University/Agency Partnership Program Preparing Students for Public Child Welfare Practice

Simple Counts (Student, Faculty, Agency Stakeholders)
Students taking child welfare classes
Students enrolled in public child welfare internships
Students accepting Title IV-E stipends
Students accepting public child welfare employment
Employees who remain beyond one year
Faculty teaching child welfare courses
Faculty including child welfare course content
Faculty attending conferences related to child welfare
Faculty conducting research in area of child welfare

Portfolios (Student, Faculty, Agency Stakeholders)
Student journals/logs
Student projects
Teaching units
Instructor journals/logs
Videotapes of classes
Videotapes of agency training

Student Self-Report Surveys (Student Stakeholders)
Satisfaction/Attitude
Pre and post awareness
Interest in child welfare
Knowledge of child welfare
Skills in child welfare
Values related to child welfare

Student Interviews (Student Stakeholders)
Pre-Internship
Beginning Internship
Mid-term Internship
Final/exit Internship

Student Performance (Student Stakeholders)
Results of competency tests on child welfare skills
Grades in child welfare courses, social work courses, overall G.P.A.
Written evaluations
Passage rate on licensure exams

Basic Skill Development Class (Student, Agency Stakeholders)
Pre and Post tests of content
Supervisor evaluation
Student evaluation of class
Student evaluation of instructors
Student self-report of learning

Longitudinal Studies of Students (Student Stakeholders)
Alumni surveys
Exit survey
Focus groups
Phone Interviews
Comparison of counts
Comparison of annual evaluations

TABLE 2 (continued)

Faculty Surveys (Faculty Stakeholders)
Staff development time related to child welfare
Amount of child welfare content included in curriculum
Research on child welfare
Addition of courses related to child welfare
Child welfare or related course enrollments
Increase in independent studies related to child welfare

Agency Surveys (Agency Stakeholder)
Satisfaction with partnership
Hiring data
Staff retention data
Quality of graduates

Comparisons of Employees Performance (Agency Stakeholder)
Social workers with non-social workers
Social workers with social workers without child welfare internship
Social workers with social workers without child welfare content or course
Social workers with stipend with social workers without stipend
Social workers with non-social workers by unit (i.e. intake, investigation, adoption)
Caseloads
Movement of worker from one job to another within agency
Time to complete tasks

Child/Family Indicators (Children/Family Stakeholders)
Baseline data on children/families compared with current data (counts)
Number of placements a child experiences
Length of time for average service
Cost of service for case
Recurrences of need for service
Quality of service as perceived by client
Quality of service as perceived by agency
Stage duration for child/family
Legal status durations (i.e. temporary management conservatorship, adoption, child emancipated)
Legal action durations (still being defined)
Placement durations
Permanency status (length of time from case opened to permanency)
Level of care for each case

bases that reveal trends in the general population, and self-comparisons over time.

Sometimes time and money constraints interfere with the gathering of information. Some universities have used e-mail surveys, conference telephone calls, distance conferencing (by interactive television or satellite) to help meet these challenges. Most partnerships find that it is both time and cost effective if the collection of information is routine and part of the normal operating routine. The key to achieving a non-invasive evaluation is to plan ahead for it and schedule it as part of the regular partnership activities.

Step 6:
Analyze Information and Use It
for Quality Improvement

Evaluations create tools for improving strategies or services and refining goals and objectives. An evaluation can show whether a program has reached its objectives and whether the failure to meet an objective was caused by inadequate implementation or flawed assumptions. This knowledge helps programs fine-tune approaches and set goals, creating a continuous loop of useful feedback. Linking the feedback to program activities on an ongoing basis allows the program to improve on a continuous basis without waiting until the end of a contract year or other specified date.

This step is important in understanding how the program is being implemented. Partnership teams will already know either from performance assessments or monitoring evaluations if the program is being accountable to its objectives (is it doing what it said it was going to do). This step is to develop a picture of the quality of what is being done. Step six is the time to examine the participants' perceptions about the program using both qualitative and quantitative data. This feedback is essential to a strong partnership.

Step 7: Examine Outcomes

This step focuses on what changes have occurred. Looking at the short-term objectives and using questionnaires, interviews, observations, performance tests, and similar measures, the evaluation is now focusing on results. What has actually happened to students who graduated from the program? Does the agency have more social workers? Is the retention rate for social workers in the agency longer than the retention rate for non-social workers? Is the performance of social workers better than the performance of non-social workers? The partnership team needs to look closely at the indicators they have chosen. The team needs to ask if the indicators present a clear picture of the outcomes of your project. If the indicators are not sufficient, the partnership team may want to begin collecting additional data.

At this point, it is often helpful to use an outcome indicator plan. A typical outcome indicator plan has four dimensions of performance measurement: quantity of effort; quality of effort; quantity of effect; and quality of effect. These four dimensions are best understood by examining them in a multidimensional grid where you look at both inputs and outputs from the perspective of both quantity and quality. The Casey Outcomes and Decision-Making Project (1998) adapted a useful model for core child welfare outcome indicators based on the earlier work of Friedman (1997).

Using their model as a guide in the case of university/agency partnerships, quantity of effort might look at program inputs such as number of courses taught and number of stipends awarded. Quality of effort might examine how well these courses were taught and by whom; it looks at the selection process for awarding stipends. Quantity of effect could report on how much content students mastered and how many stipend recipients were hired. Quality of effect might present improved scores on licensing or competency exams; it might highlight the number of promotions or merit awards for students educated in the partnership program. Depending of the goals of the partnership, these four indicators can be translated to efforts or effects on different constituencies. Some partnerships focus on outcomes for the stipend students; others focus on outcomes for the children and families who are the recipients of the services of these newly prepared child welfare workers.

Step 8: Assess Impact/Cost-effectiveness

Assessing long-term impact follows the examination of outcomes. This is point where the partnership team will need a rigorous research design, including a comparison group. How the team designs an impact study depends on time, money, and the results of the outcome studies. There is a dearth of impact studies in the field, and it may be to the partnership's advantage to link with other programs in order to have a larger sample and more resources than the team would have using only one program.

To examine cost effectiveness, one university/agency partnership has calculated the cost savings to the agency when it does not have to hire new employees because of a lowered turnover rate. Another partnership (where social work students who have completed internships in the child protective service agency are hired upon graduation) has calculated the cost savings for having students prepared in internships and ready to go to work for the child welfare agency as a three month saving (training time and cost for new employees). Another university computes the months of service to the child protective services agency beyond the student's contractual commitment for repayment. Each partnership needs to find ways to examine impact and cost effectiveness.

These eight steps can be a guide for programs and partnerships. It is important to remember that the evaluation process is not linear. Evaluators must loop backward in order to move forward. Systematic periodic assessment of who the stakeholders are, the efficacy of service improvement strategies, goal and objective clarifications, and other modifications need to be made along the way to examining outcomes. An example of this recently occurred at step 2 "clarify the goal" for one program. The team was writing out goal statements and realized that many of the goals of the partnership included changes at the training unit level, but they had not included the agency trainers as stakeholders. The team went back to step one and identify agency trainers to include on the team and in the evaluation planning process. It is essential that feedback occur at each step of the evaluation process. Partnerships are living entities and often need to make revisions and adjust their plans based on the findings at each new step. Some authors have called this stage "needs assessment," but we have found that needs assessment is a process and is ongoing. It is not just one step in the evaluation process because needs keep changing. These beginning steps are a tool and not a fixed product; each partnership must adapt and use them as appropriate.

EVALUATION ISSUES

Most university/agency partnerships recognize that evaluations should be an important part of their program, but these same partnerships usually list a variety of reasons why they don't have a comprehensive evaluation plan in place. Knowledge, time and budget constraints are key factors that influence the ability of a partnership program to develop and conduct evaluations.

Evaluation is essential to university/agency partnerships. The field is always changing, and partnership teams must use evaluation as a tool to keep abreast of what is happening in the field of child welfare, in social work education, and in public sector social work. The rules change, the students change, the faculty change, the agency administrators change; everything changes. This field is so dynamic that one can't possibly predict what lies ahead. The only way to keep abreast and be able to forecast some of what the future holds is to have a built-in evaluation process for all components of the university/agency partnership. Evaluation is the key to the success of what university/agency partnerships are doing. If partnership teams assess progress, then they are able to answer the accountability questions from university, federal, and state administrators. Partnership teams are able to tell what has happened already and where they are heading.

Future studies need to be undertaken, and these studies need to extend beyond case examples to include large samples of university/agency partnership programs. The studies need be conducted on a systematic basis by gathering both written and interview data from the projects. Budgets also need to be examined. Although the overall budget for most programs can easily be determined, it is often difficult to determine how much money is specifically allocated to evaluation.

Critical problems persist and need to be the subject of future research: How do we know if university/agency partnerships to prepare students for public child welfare are working? How can evaluations control for extraneous variables such as workplace climate or a freeze in job hiring? How can evaluations control for individual variables (personality, attitude, prior knowledge)? How do we determine if one partnership's approach is better than another is? Which partnerships are cost-effective? How can we link child welfare training to quality issues such as fewer cases of child abuse/neglect?

RECOMMENDATIONS

It is important for partnerships to keep several recommendations in mind when designing their evaluations. First, be clear about the outcomes you are seeking. After you have identified your key stakeholders, make certain that all are in agreement about the goals of the university/agency partnership. It is critical to specify early on what results you are seeking with the partnership effort. University/agency partnerships must involve participants in the partnership evaluation. Designing the evaluation collaboratively and sharing the role of expert are essential. Starting from the "bottom up" helps the researcher understand what is happening in the partnership and receive constructive criticism of the measures and the process being used to collect data.

Other recommendations include isolating the specific components of the partnership in your evaluation in order to examine more fully the role that each part plays in the partnership. For example, it is important to know how well the courses are being taught and how well the internship experience is working. Using objective measures rather than self-report measures whenever possible will strengthen the evaluation. The limitations on reliability and validity of self-report measures compromise the research on partnerships. In addition to some standardized measures, direct observation can be helpful in counting interactions and documenting behavioral changes. Gomby and Larson (1992) recognize that many partnerships focus on changes in attitudes but caution that changes in attitudes don't always lead to changes in behaviors. They suggest that although self-report paper-and-pencil surveys are easy, they are not always the most predictive of changes. Keir and Millea (1997) caution that programs should not collect data just because it is available. The data may not be closely linked to the outcomes. Partnerships need to be clear about the outcomes they are seeking when they select measures and clearly link the measures to the outcomes they are seeking.

CONCLUSION

In sum, evaluation should be a key component of all child welfare partnerships; evaluation should be a key focus for both individual programs that the partnership sponsors and the partnership as a whole. Unless we include evaluation as a critical component of university/agency partnerships to prepare students for public child welfare, we will continue to produce inadequate evaluations that do not serve the purposes for which they are intended. Evaluations that are not integral parts of child welfare partnerships from the beginning will be evaluations in name only. The eight steps discussed here are beginning steps to help universities and child welfare agencies think about their goals and what they want to accomplish with the dollars they are receiving from federal or state funding. University/agency partnerships must meet the challenge and take a new look at what they are evaluating and how they are evaluating their programs, their activities, and their partnerships. Evaluation of these complex partnerships is not an easy task, but it can be done. We will better serve children, families, students, universities, and agencies if we improve our evaluation studies.

REFERENCES

Alperin, D. E. (1998). Factors relating to student satisfaction with child welfare field placements. *Journal of Social Work Education, 34(1),* 43-54.

Alter, C. & Murty, S. (1997). Logic modeling: A tool for teaching practice evaluation. *Journal of Social Work Education, 33,* 103-117.

Baer, B. & McLean, A. (1994). *A report: Child welfare curriculum in accredited BSW programs.* Green Bay: University of Wisconsin Social Work Program.

Casey Outcomes and Decision-Making Project. (1998). *Assessing outcomes in child welfare services: Principles, concepts, and a framework of core indicators.* Englewood, CO: author.

Dryfoos, J. (1994). *Full-service schools: A revolution in health and social services for children, youth, and families.* San Francisco, CA: Jossey-Bass.

Freeman, E. M. & Pennekamp, M. (1988). *Social work practice: Toward a child, family, school, community perspective.* Springfield, IL: Charles C. Thomas.

Friedman, M. (1997). *A guide to developing and using performance measures in results-based budgeting.* Washington, DC: The Finance Project.

Gabor, P. A., Unrau, Y. A., & Grinnell, R. M., Jr. (1998). *Evaluation for social workers: A quality improvement approach for the social services.* Boston: Allyn & Bacon.

Gomby, D. S. & Larson, C. S. (1992). Evaluation of school linked services. *The Future of Children, 2(1),* 68-84.

Hooper-Briar, K. & Larson, H. A. (1994). *Serving children, youth and families through interprofessional collaboration and service integration.* Oxford, OH: The Danforth Foundation and The Institute for Educational Renewal at Miami University.

Jacobs, F., Hrusa Williams, P., Kapuscik, H., & Kates, E. (1998). *Evaluating family preservation services: A guide for state administrators.* Medford, MA: Family Preservation Evaluation Project, Tufts University.

Keir, S. S. & Millea, S. (1997). *Challenges and realities: Evaluating a school-based service project*. Austin, TX: Hogg Foundation for Mental Health.

Knapp, M. S. (1995). How shall we study comprehensive, collaborative services for children and families? *Educational Researcher, 24(4)*, 5-16.

Leighninger, L. & Ellett, A. J. (1998). De-professionalization in child welfare: Historical Analysis and implications for social work education. Paper presented at Council on Social Work Education 44th Annual Program Meeting, Orlando, Florida, March 5-8.

Lieberman, A. A., Hornby, H., & Russell, M. (1988). Educational backgrounds and work experiences of child welfare personnel. *Social Work, 33*, 485-489.

Melaville, A. I. & Blank, M. J. (1993). *Together we can: A guide for crafting a profamily system of education and human services*. Washington, DC: U. S. Government Printing Office.

Rome, S. (1994). Choosing child welfare: An analysis of social work students' career choices. Washington, DC: National Association of Social Workers.

Rossi, P. H.,Freeman, H. E., Lipsey, M. (1998). *Evaluation: A systematic approach*. 6th ed. Newbury Park, CA: Sage Publications.

Royse, D. & Thyer, B. A. (2000). *Program evaluation: An introduction*. Chicago: Nelson-Hall.

Weiss, H. B. & Greene, J. G. (1992). An empowerment partnership for family support and education programs and evaluation. *Family Science Review, 5(1)*, 131-148.

Weiss, H. & Jacobs, F.(Eds.) (1988). *Evaluating family programs*. Hawthorne, NY: Aldine de Gruyter.

Zlotnik, J. L. (1997). *Preparing the workforce for family-centered practice: Social work education and public human services partnerships*. Alexandria, VA: Council on Social Work Education.

Finding and Keeping Child Welfare Workers: Effective Use of Training and Professional Development

Stephen R. Fox

Viola P. Miller

Anita P. Barbee

SUMMARY. Administrators in public human services are constantly involved in the exhausting challenge of recruiting and training staff in the child welfare arena. This article describes a program that the Commonwealth of Kentucky developed in order to address the recruitment and retention issue. The Public Child Welfare Certification Program is a special multi-university preparation program designed to recruit excellent workers from BSW programs who are prepared to take on complex cases with normal supervision within weeks of employment and to sus-

Stephen R. Fox, MSW, is affiliated with the University Training Consortium, Eastern Kentucky University.

Viola P. Miller, EdD, is affiliated with Cabinet for Families and Children, Commonwealth of Kentucky.

Anita P. Barbee, PhD, is affiliated with The Kent School of Social Work, University of Louisville.

Address correspondence to: Anita P. Barbee, PhD, Kent School of Social Work, University of Louisville, Louisville, KY 40292 (E-mail: anita.barbee@louisville.edu) or to Stephen R. Fox, MSW, University Training Consortium, Eastern Kentucky University, 300 Stratton Building, 521 Lancaster Avenue, Richmond, KY 40475 (E-mail: trcfox@acs.eku.edu).

[Haworth co-indexing entry note]: "Finding and Keeping Child Welfare Workers: Effective Use of Training and Professional Development." Fox, Stephen R. Viola P. Miller, and Anita P. Barbee. Co-published simultaneously in *Journal of Human Behavior in the Social Environment* (The Haworth Social Work Practice Press, an imprint of The Haworth Press, Inc.) Vol. 7, No. 1/2, 2003, pp. 67-81; and: *Charting the Impacts of University-Child Welfare Collaboration* (ed: Katharine Briar-Lawson, and Joan Levy Zlotnik) The Haworth Social Work Practice Press, an imprint of The Haworth Press, Inc., 2003, pp. 67-81. Single or multiple copies of this article are available for a fee from The Haworth Document Delivery Service [1-800-HAWORTH, 9:00 a.m. - 5:00 p.m. (EST). E-mail address: getinfo@haworthpressinc.com].

tain those workers over time. Evaluation of the pilot indicates that the program is a great success in preparing students for child welfare work. Implications are discussed. *[Article copies available for a fee from The Haworth Document Delivery Service: 1-800-HAWORTH. E-mail address: <getinfo@haworthpressinc.com> Website: <http://www.HaworthPress.com> © 2003 by The Haworth Press, Inc. All rights reserved.]*

KEYWORDS. Child welfare, recruitment and retention, BSW education

What began as a practical initiative to better prepare potential public child welfare workers may hold the key for solving a major part of the age-old problem of recruitment and retention. The employee recruitment and retention issue has exploded on the corporate scene and has grabbed and held the attention of top-level CEO's and their human resources staff ever since the jobless rate began its decline to 4% (ASTD, 2000). Studies in the corporate sector have found that training and professional development are a key aspect of recruiting and retaining talented workers (ASTD, 2000). Compared to the average company, top companies in this arena provide more training, spend more as a percentage of payroll on training, use more learning technologies and less classroom training, utilize more outside resources for training, concentrate on human services management practices and select employees very carefully (ASTD, 2000). One point of particular significance was that these companies do not pay huge signing bonuses or exorbitant salaries, a common practice among other organizations involved in the talent wars. On the contrary, these companies count heavily on their positive, employee-centered culture to attract and keep employees. This does not mean that they do not pay competitive salaries. It does mean that they understand that it is not just money that drives recruitment and retention.

Implications for Child Welfare Recruitment and Retention

Administrators in public human services are constantly involved in the exhausting challenge of recruiting and retaining staff in the child welfare arena. There is no more challenging, stressful and thankless job in the public sector than that of the public child welfare worker. The long hours, the physical threats, the stress of dealing day in and day out with families and children in crisis take a terrible toll on these workers. It is often said that they "burn out" after about a year on the job. Experiences as front line workers and in administration of a public social services agency actually contradict this belief.

Workers *don't* decide to leave the job after a year. Most workers (especially child protective services workers) make this decision within the first one or two months of employment and in some cases even sooner. In many instances these new, energetic, enthusiastic workers are overwhelmed the day they walk into the office. Their welcoming ceremony is often a stack of case records that have been sitting on the empty desk of the "former" worker. The exuberant statements of "O wow! Am I glad to see you! We are just about to die. Your position has been vacant for three months!" tells the new worker that they are welcome but also hints of the chaos that may exist in the office. They are sent to training early on but often have been overwhelmed by the tasks already assigned.

About four years ago, one author ran into Mary, a former BSW student of his from a university where he is an adjunct professor. Quite frankly, she looked terrible! She was participating in her first core competency training for the agency. After exchanging some pleasantries he asked her when she joined the agency and how she was doing. This young woman, whom he remembered from class as energetic, creative and very upbeat, had changed dramatically. She told him that she had been on the job about one month and was already looking for another job. He gently remarked that she looked exhausted. She responded that, "I am. I am totally worn out and very unhappy." He asked her why. She responded that her job was not what she expected and that she already had forty ongoing child protective services cases assigned to her and didn't know where to start. She said that coming to this training was great because it gave her a way to escape from the office for a while but that she also knew that things would be worse when she returned. She went on to say that she was going to try and make her six-months probation and then try to transfer to another area. He really did not know what to say to the young person. She was clearly one of the brightest and energy filled student in her class in college but now carried all of the signs of burnout after only one month on the job!

Was this perhaps an isolated incident of a young worker that had chosen the wrong profession or at least the wrong part of her profession? This was not the case. Four years later with the experience of a new and innovative program to better prepare workers for public child welfare service we all realized that Mary's situation was not unique. Comments from students completing training confirmed that many new employees in the system were overwhelmed. They were often oppressed not only by the workload but also by the crisis driven environment of casework and lack of a sense of personal or professional value.

Combining the understanding of early burn out with the recent data on retention in the corporate sector provides interesting and critical data for dealing with these issues in child welfare.

Recruitment and Retention–Old Issue/New Approaches

Actions by the Kentucky Cabinet for Families and Children and its University Training Consortium over the past four years have established a strategy that is beginning to have a positive impact on recruitment and retention (Fox, Burnham, & Miller, 1997). This effort has been supported by Title IV-E training funds.

This approach is based upon the data presented above on organizational development. Cabinet Secretary Viola Miller, a former Dean of Continuation Education and Academic Outreach, at Murray State University, has established a significant strategy for changing the culture of the agency and dramatically improving performance. She and her management team have established three elements as targets for cultural change that in turn will lead to the creation of the learning organization. This cultural change can greatly enhance the agency's employee recruitment and retention activities. This movement is also an integral part of Kentucky governor Paul Patton's Empower Kentucky Program that is revitalizing and improving Kentucky's government operations.

The three elements that are the key principals for improvement are: create a culture that values the employee, create a learning organization based upon mission, vision and outcomes, and implement true learning transfer and reinforcement. Institutionalizing these three elements directly relates to the agency's focus on recruiting and retaining child welfare staff.

The activities of the Cabinet for Families and the University Training Consortium (eight public universities in partnership with each other and with the Cabinet) in these three areas are aimed at enhancing not only the accomplishment of the goals of the agency but to create a culture that will successful recruit the brightest and most dedicated workers and keep them for their entire career.

Making Recruitment and Retention Work–Creation of the Kentucky Public Child Welfare Certification Program

As part of the creation of the learning organization, the Kentucky Cabinet for Families and Children and its university partners have developed a unique pre-employment program: The Public Child Welfare Certification Program. This special multi-university preparation program was designed to recruit excellent workers who are prepared to take on complex cases with normal supervision within weeks (rather than months) of employment and to sustain those workers over time.

In 1996, administrators in the Cabinet for Families and Children wanted to do more to prepare BSW students to work in the public child welfare sector.

While most social work students across the country are receiving excellent preparation as generalists, public child welfare administrators are in immediate need of competent workers who in a very short time can effectively carry cases. This tension of need versus availability is not a new issue. What is new is Kentucky's social work education community and the public agency's approach to solving the problem. In the past, universities and agencies have had little success in dealing with the issue. The universities view skill development (which the agency wants) as totally foreign to their academic mission. In a superb example of effective dialogue and problem solving in Kentucky, the two entities created a legitimate process that would satisfy the program needs of the agency and at the same time enhance the academic quality of course work with a commitment to the academic mission of the university.

Secretary Miller was already beginning to formulate her vision for the creation of a cultural change in the agency and the formation of the learning organization. It was rather ironic that Steve Fox, a career social services practitioner was leaving the public agency for the university sector and the secretary was leaving the university sector coming to the public human services arena. Several meetings occurred to discuss the role of the University Training Consortium and its long time role in training and professional development services for the Cabinet. Part of those discussions centered on the idea of an agency/university partnership to address the issue of pre-employment preparation of child welfare workers.

Doug Burnham, the director of the Eastern Kentucky University Social Work program, and a highly respected member and leader of the Kentucky Association of Social Work Educators was briefed on the issue of advanced preparation for child welfare workers through the social work baccalaureate programs. He also saw value in pursuing the concept and was instrumental in communicating the concept to the other members of the Association. In early April of 1996, Secretary Miller and Steve Fox met with the Association and the Secretary extended an open invitation to partner with the agency in creating the new learning culture. This group, along with staff of the agency and with the University Training Consortium acting as staff and support, began work on the Public Child Welfare Certification Program.

Structure and Work of the Design Team

With a mission to design and implement a creative process to advance the education and performance of potential BSW front-line child welfare workers, a special design committee was formed. Participants included directors and faculty of nine social work programs, representatives of program staff from the Cabinet for Families and Children, a representative from distance learning technology, training faculty from the Cabinet, a representative of the Cabinet's personnel office and the Director of the University Training Consortium.

This group met once a month for approximately one year to design the program. The committee was co-chaired by the director of the EKU Social Work Program and the director of the UTC. The most impressive aspect of the design period was the collaboration between all of the universities and the training personnel of the Cabinet. While there was healthy dialogue and periodic professional disagreement on issues, there was no sign of any turf problems. On the contrary, as the final plan for a pilot program reflects, the highest level of partnership collaboration was evident.

This team designed the preliminary model for the Public Child Welfare Certification Program. The design consisted of the following: two elective child welfare courses to address practice and theory, a jointly designed common syllabus for each course, common tests and common texts, shared faculty, use of agency trainers as adjunct faculty for portions of the courses, intense field practicums in public child welfare offices, completion of agency competency training before graduation, tuition and stipends for selected students, entry into the agency system at a higher classification level and a two year employment commitment.

The fact that nine universities and the state agency trainers could agree on common syllabi, tests and texts and shared instructors was considered rather revolutionary and amazing. For those of us who understood the long history of partnerships among Kentucky university social work programs and the public agency there was no shock. The fact the IV-E Funded University Training Consortium had for over ten years been the training support, development and delivery partner with the child welfare portion of the Cabinet also contributed to the relative ease with which the collaboration occurred.

The Student Participants

Critical decisions about the process of program implementation were paramount. After much discussion it was decided to pilot the program in universities that volunteered. It was further decided that each participating university would select (along with the agency) five students at the junior or senior level for participation.

The design team prepared a detailed student selection process that would be later used at the participating universities. That process included a written application, 3 letters of recommendation, selection criteria (including an overall GPA of 2.5, a 3.0 GPA in all social work courses, at least three semesters of undergraduate study left to complete, completion of a social work practice course), and joint university/agency interviews. The writers of the recommendations are asked to rate the candidates on a 1 (limited) to 5 (high) scale on such dimensions as level of maturity and emotional stability, understanding of self, sensitivity to the needs and feelings of others, ability to respect and work with differences in people, oral communication skills, verbal communication skills, ability to work with others and ability to accept constructive feedback. Applicants strengths and weaknesses are detailed and recommendation with enthusiasm to non-recommendation is then made. The interview focuses on the applicant's exploration into the public child welfare field, the source of their motivation, their interpersonal behavior and manner, their sense of accountability to a job, pertinent aspects of their background and overall assessment of the candidate.

It was agreed that the state agency would pay full tuition for the participants as well as a stipend for expenses. In addition, the students who successfully completed the program would be hired into the agency at a higher classification level. In turn the student signed a contract that he or she would work two years for the agency. Any student who does not complete the program or does not accept employment with the agency must pay back all of the money received during the program including tuition.

In addition to the two electives, special practicum with the agency and attendance at special faculty/agency/student retreats, the students must complete the core competency agency training immediately prior to graduation.

The Pilot–Two Years of Excitement and Learning

In the fall of 1997, 30 undergraduate students at six universities began the pursuit of certification in public child welfare. The universities involved in the pilot program were Eastern Kentucky University, Morehead State University, Murray State University, Northern Kentucky University, Spalding University, and the University of Kentucky. The University of Louisville provided the outcome evaluation for the project.

During the following two years, faculty, agency training staff, and students focused on the ultimate goal of the program–the in-depth preparation of undergraduate social work students for public child welfare employment. The students had been selected following screening and competitive interviews by university and agency personnel. The common syllabi for the two courses had been prepared after hours of discussion and planning by the design team of university faculty and agency trainers. The interactive television departments of each university had made preparations for the simultaneous broadcast of classes at each university. The students were in the process of receiving a stipend check at the beginning of each semester and each university was receiving full tuition payments for each student through the primary IV-E contractor, Eastern Kentucky University.

For two years the students learned in the classroom, biannual retreats and intense, specially designed practicums. At the end of their program (last semester) they attended the core competency training for new employees of the Cabinet for Families and Children.

At the same time the faculty, agency trainers and university/agency design group also learned. As the director of the Murray State University social work program said, "It is hard to believe that after a full year of strategic planning we would still have so many new questions and issues two weeks after the program began!" It seemed that every week new issues arose that demanded attention of the design group–student contract language concerning requirements, probation status for a students who's GPA in social work courses had dropped, technology difficulties in putting together six universities, confusion over how to cover the agency core competency training and still complete the class requirements of the university, and many others issues!

The group quickly realized the efficacy in piloting and evaluating the program with only one cohort of students before planning a long-term continuation. With each new issue or problem the team became more confident in problem solving and administering the program. However, process evaluation results lead to numerous changes in operations.

EVALUATION METHOD

There was a process evaluation and an outcome evaluation of the program. The process evaluation was conducted by a PCWCP faculty member at the University of Kentucky. The faculty member attended all meetings, taught a class for the program and interviewed students, coordinators, faculty and Cabinet trainers and administrators in order to capture the program's processes and feelings about those processes.

The outcome evaluation on the first cohort of participants in the program was conducted by the Kent School of Social Work at the University of Louisville, one of the eight public universities in the Kentucky University Training Consortium. Twenty-seven students in the cohort included 14% males and 86% females. Three students who began the program did not complete the program due to personal issues.

The evaluation contained two components: (1) A comparison of the pre and post-test scores of PCWCP students with the scores of other new employees completing the agency core competency training and (2) The results of structured interviews with graduates and their supervisors six months after the completion of their education.

As was mentioned above, all students in the program were required to complete the agency core competency training for new employees prior to graduation. These trainings cover approximately five weeks spread out over three months (PCWCP students are exempted from those modules that are identical to their course work). All participants were required to complete pre and post-tests for the courses. The pre-post tests included 69 multiple-choice items that related directly to the course objectives and content. The participants were graded based on the percent of items that were correct.

The structured interviews involved both rating scales and open-ended questions. The survey instrument was based upon 26 formal "behavioral anchors" identified within the core competency training that must be present before new employees can carry child welfare cases. These 26 anchors were the foundational elements for the agency/university designed training transfer system in Kentucky (Barbee et al., in press). Each PCWCP graduate and supervisor was asked to rate the graduates as they compared with other new workers on the 26 areas using the scale 1(substandard) 2(below average) 3(average) 4(above average) and 5(superior). The 26 behaviors dealt with a variety of competencies in child welfare practice from skills in communication and appropriate professional behavior to skills in case assessment and planning. The specific behaviors included: attitude, relationships, safety and permanency planning. In addition, the new worker's abilities were rated in terms of best practices in skills such as intake, investigations, ongoing treatment, court behaviors, and others were measured (see Table 1 for descriptions of each behavior rated and the results for both graduates and their supervisors).

In addition, both graduates and supervisors rated on a 1 (not at all) to 5 (a great deal) the extent to which they recommended that the program continue, the likelihood of hiring other PCWCP graduates and the extent to which they recommended the program to others.

The open-ended questions for supervisors asked about why the program should or should not be continued, how the program could be improved and to recommend any knowledge or particular skill set that should be included in future PCWCP classes. Graduates were asked these same questions as well as what specific knowledge and skills taught in the program helped them in their work with the Cabinet.

TABLE 1. Means and Standard Deviations of the Supervisor and Self Ratings on 26 Job Skills for the PCWCP Students

	Supervisor Ratings		Self Ratings	
	Mean	S.D.	Mean	S.D.
Attitude towards superiors	4.35	1.02	4.31	.84
Attitude towards social work	4.56	.65	-----	
Relationship with clients	4.28	.84	4.46	.81
Relationship with ethnic minorities	4.27	.70	4.23	.71
Relationship with agencies	3.88	.73	4.19	.85
Joining with clients	4.25	.74	4.50	.76
Dealing with resistant clients	3.92	.97	4.04	.96
Utilizing the permanency planning goal	3.74	.54	4.27	.72
Remaining safe and disease free	4.23	.69	4.23	.86
Asking appropriate questions during Intake	4.30	1.03	4.31	1.35
Demonstrating knowledge of criteria for referrals	4.18	.80	4.19	.75
Remaining respectful during referral process	4.32	.78	4.56	.65
Demonstrating knowledge of appropriate time frames for investigations	4.30	.63	4.52	.71
Demonstrating knowledge and skills in child development	4.09	1.00	4.08	.81
Demonstrating knowledge of parenting strategies	4.08	1.02	3.88	.73
Can identify dynamics and indicators of abuse and neglect	4.08	.80	4.56	.58
Can conduct a risk assessment and make accurate determinations	4.05	.85	4.24	.78
Demonstrating knowledge of dynamics and indicators of domestic violence	4.09	.75	4.48	.77
Demonstrating knowledge of the effects of domestic violence on children in the home	4.16	.85	4.40	.82
Demonstrating knowledge of the dynamics and indicators of child sexual abuse	3.77	1.18	4.36	.81
Demonstrating knowledge of the particular strategies to investigate child sexual abuse	3.69	1.77	4.00	1.08

	Supervisor Ratings		Self Ratings	
	Mean	S.D.	Mean	S.D.
Can write a case assessment utilizing family level and individual level patterns and issues	3.95	.90	4.12	1.01
Can write a case plan utilizing the solution-based casework	3.86	.91	4.00	1.58
Demonstrating the knowledge of the law and the use of legal documents	3.83	.70	3.36	.81
Demonstrating competent courtroom Preparation and behavior	3.95	.72	4.20	91
Demonstrating ability to close a case	4.15	.90	4.04	1.10

EVALUATION RESULTS

Process Evaluation Results

It was clear to the faculty and agency staff that something very special was beginning to happen during the pilot project. The following overarching results were found from the process evaluation: (1) The faculty of the six universities became closer due to the tremendous energy that they were expending in developing and implementing the program. (2) Faculty and agency staff were working closely and gaining a deeper appreciation for each other. (3) Faculty, agency representatives, and students were beginning a real bonding process especially through the two, day and one-half retreats each year of the program. (4) Agency staff were making very positive statements about the students' performance during their practicums. (5) Everyone involved with the program was beginning to feel that they "were on the road to something very exciting and positive." (6) All six universities were excited about the potential of the program. Three of them realized a special value in their regions. Northern Kentucky University (metropolitan Cincinnati, Ohio) was beginning to see the program as a means of addressing the recruitment and retention issue in this major population area where competition was fierce. Morehead State University (the north-eastern Appalachian region of Kentucky) saw the program as a "shot in the arm" for child welfare services in the Appalachian section. Spalding University (the only private University in the Pilot) became a major supplier of BSW employees for the largest Cabinet for Families and Children region in the state.

The pilot was extremely successful. In addition to the concrete data of the report, the two-year pilot demonstrated the fact that multiple universities cannot only "co-exist" but can collaborate in a manner and to an extent rarely witnessed. Experts in higher education still marvel at the fact that six universities (actually nine when you count the design team) could agree on identical syllabi, common texts and tests and share faculty through the use of interactive television and internet communication channels. Another "outcome" of the pilot not captured in the formal evaluation was the strong bond that formed between university faculty, agency staff and students. This bonding was obvious during the retreats. The building of strong mentoring relationships that can endure over time will be an unintended consequence of the Public Child Welfare Certification Program.

Outcome Evaluation Results

When the pre-post scores of the PCWCP 27 students were compared to a randomly chosen cohort of 27 students who took the training and the tests at the same time as the PCWCP students, it was found that the PCWCP students scored significantly higher on both tests than the other new employees. The PCWCP students moved from a mean of 48.6 on the pre-test to a mean of 52.6 on the post-test ($t(23) = 7.19$, $p < .0001$), while the other trainees improved ($t(25) = 7.38$, $p < .01$) but both began at a lower level (Pre-Mean = 42.8) and ended at a lower level (Post-Mean = 48.5) than did PCWCP trainees. The PCWCP graduates were higher than other trainees in undergraduate GPA (Means = 3.39 vs. 3.13, respectively), but when this variable was taken into account in the comparison of groups, the PCWCP group still performed better in training than did the non-PCWCP group ($F(2,38) = 3.22$, $p < .08$). This finding is significant in that it indicates that the intense concentration of both theory and practice in the classroom and in the practicum produced what appears to be a stronger transfer of learning than perhaps that which is available in the traditional academic classes.

It also says something to the fact that these special students have had a concentration of learning related to child welfare over a period of three semesters whereas the other new employees (especially those without a social work degree) were only getting a concentration of learning for a five week period.

The most significant results of the evaluation were the outcomes for the graduates on the job as indicated on the structured interviews of both supervisors and graduates. The results were outstanding and confirmed the expectations of the faculty and agency staff.

The supervisors rated the new graduates' behavior very high with an overall average of 4.1 on the 5-point scale ($s.d. = .86$) for each of the behaviors listed in Table 1. The Cabinet and the universities were particularly interested in the ranking of the workers in the areas of intake, investigation and treatment. Those scores were as follows: Intake ($M = 4.30$, $s.d. = .87$), Investigations ($M =$

4.0, *s.d.* = .98), Ongoing treatment (*M* = 4.0, *s.d.* = .91), Court related behaviors (*M* = 3.97, *s.d.* = .71).

In general, agency supervisors considered the graduates to be: better prepared to handle complex cases much sooner (months!) than other new employees including BSW graduates, less stressed and much more confident, more skilled in interacting with clients, more knowledgeable of agency policy and procedures and, much more positive in their attitudes about the agency and their job.

The supervisors recommended that the program continue (*M* = 4.80, *s.d.* = .50), indicated that they would be likely to hire another PCWCP graduate if the opportunity arose (*M* = 4.88, *s.d.* = .45) and would highly recommend that other supervisors hire graduates of the PCWCP program (*M* = 4.84, *s.d.* = .47).

The PCWCP graduates also rated themselves very high on the 26 behavioral anchors with an average of 4.22 on the 5-point scale (*s.d.* = .87). The scores on the sub-areas included: Intake (*M* = 4.35, *s.d.* = .92), Investigations (*M* = 4.26, *s.d.* = .81), Ongoing treatment (*M* = 4.0, *s.d.* = 1.58), Court related behaviors (*M* = 3.86, *s.d.* = .86).

The graduates of the PCWCP program gave the following reactions to the program: This program was essential for preparation for such a complicated job; they would have felt overwhelmed without the knowledge and skills they gained in the program. This program provided them with the knowledge and skills to work with clients. Coming out of such an intensive program, they felt more competent to carry a caseload and much less stressed than other new workers they observed. Networking during their field placement and training experience helped them understand the Cabinet better and provided them with a network of support once the job started. They believe they will not burnout or leave the agency as a result of their preparation for the job through the program.

The graduates recommended that the program continue (*M* = 4.70, *s.d.* = .76), recommended that other students participate in the PCWCP program (*M* = 4.65, *s.d.* = .88), recommended that supervisors hire graduates of the PCWCP program (*M* = 4.78, *s.d.* = .67) and believed that the PCWCP prepared them for their job with the Cabinet (*M* = 4.78, *s.d.* = .79).

Further follow-up presentations by graduates at later retreats confirmed that they felt that the PCWCP had prepared them very well for their work. More than one graduate indicated that if they had not clearly understood the demands of the child welfare position that they received through the PCWCP they would have been looking for a job immediately after their probation period. They also indicated that they had already seen other new workers come and leave after a few weeks because of the overwhelming demands of the work.

Current Status of the Program

Following a review of the positive outcomes of the pilot program, the Secretary of the Cabinet for Families and Children approved the implementation of the PCWCP as the primary, ongoing agency process for recruitment and preparation of all child welfare employees. As a result of this approval, the Secretary increased the number of slots from five per university to ten. As of September 2000 there are now nine universities in the program with an upper limit of ten students per university and the University of Louisville continues to evaluate the program. (Kentucky State University, Western Kentucky University and Brescia College were added to the program). The Secretary has also indicated that the programs should be expanded to produce as many graduates as possible.

The university/agency partnership continues to learn and change. The addition of the three universities has stretched the technology requirements to the limits. Difficulties with on line operation are monitored closely and changes are being made. For example, during the pilot the two classroom hours were totally on interactive television. The program now contains approximately one hour of interactive television linking the nine universities and one hour of class work within each university. This has maintained the interconnectivity of all of the universities but also allows for concentration on application and practice of the material.

Where adherence to payback requirements was rather liberal during the pilot (because of the numerous changes) these requirements are being strictly enforced in the ongoing program. The selection process has been strengthened for the ongoing program based upon issues discovered during the pilot program. More contact through the use of the internet is being employed and discussed. A list-serve for all faculty has been established and has proven to be an extremely useful communication tool. Another list–serve for students has been established but is not working as well as was expected.

The faculty/agency/student retreats continue to be one of the most valuable parts of the program. In addition, each year a pre-session retreat is held for all new students where former students attend to answer questions, encourage and support them.

The Future

Evaluation of the first cohorts of the PCWCP is proving that what started as a practical initiative to gain qualified staff for the field holds the potential for aggressively addressing the issue of recruitment of competent staff that can "hit the ground running." It also provides the opportunity for professionalization of the child welfare staff in states that do not require a BSW for entry-level workers.

The evaluation of the program's impact on retention is just beginning since a number of the original graduates are completing their two-year employment commitment to the agency. The agency and university partners will be closely watching the outcome of this evaluation for its potential impact on retention.

Another positive implication of the PCWCP is the potential for the development of multi-university partnerships focusing on a practical win/win initiative. (Five states are currently looking a the possibility of replicating the PCWCP.) Kentucky has had a long history of inter-university cooperation and collaboration. This is not always the case in all states. The replication of the PCWCP or a similar model could be the catalyst for establishing or enhancing similar partnerships in those places where turfism hinders positive collaboration.

If the organizational development experts are correct and the establishment of a positive work culture based upon the development of the "learning organization" will result in effective recruitment and retention programs, then we are on the right track.

The story of "Mary, the overwhelmed worker" would have been far different had the PCWCP program been in existence. The level of work shocked Mary, she lacked confidence, and she was clearly not ready to work. After one month she was looking for another position or a way out of the agency. Graduates of the PCWCP consistently report that they are prepared to face the challenges of front-line child welfare work. They speak about having more confidence and are not surprised by the scope of the work. Supervisors describe them as having personal traits of confidence and enthusiasm. They are organized, objective and professional. They demonstrate calmness in the face of difficult situations and clients.

The implementation of a pre-employment preparation process involving multiple universities in partnership with the public agency is a major step in recruitment, preparation and retention of the "best" child welfare workers. The "at risk" families and children of our nation deserve nothing less.

REFERENCES

American Society of Training and Development (2000). *Recruiting and retaining employees: Using training and education in the war for talent. A consortium benchmarking study by ASTD and SHRM*. Washington D. C.: Author.

Barbee, A.P., Yankelor, P.A., Antle, B.F., Fox, S.R., Harman, D., Evans, S.L. & Black, P. (in press). Same title. *Childwelfare*.

Fox, S. R., Burnham, D., & Miller, V. P. (1997). Reengineering the child welfare training and professional development system in Kentucky. *Public Welfare, 55*, 8-13.

Preparing for Child Welfare Practice: Themes, a Cognitive-Affective Model, and Implications from a Qualitative Study

Daniel Coleman
Sherrill Clark

SUMMARY. Specialized child welfare MSW programs and stipend support for child welfare MSW students have been developed in several states through the Federal Title IV-E program. Thirty-seven focus groups conducted over four years with approximately 550 Title IV-E MSW students in California were submitted to qualitative thematic analysis. The intense emotional challenge of child welfare work emerged in the focus groups. A three stage cognitive-affective model of student development is proposed. This exploratory study suggests several hypotheses for further research: that students at more advanced cognitive-affective levels should be less prone to burnout, better able to make the difficult value-based decisions demanded by child welfare work, and more likely to integrate and use the emotions of themselves and others. Im-

Daniel Coleman, PhD, MSW, is Assistant Professor, School of Social Work, Boston University.

Sherrill Clark, PhD, is Executive Director, California Social Work Education Center, (CalSWEC), School of Social Welfare, University of California, Berkeley.

Address correspondence to: Daniel Coleman, Boston University, School of Social Work, 264 Bay State Road, Boston, MA 02215 (E-mail: coleman1@bu.edu).

[Haworth co-indexing entry note]: "Preparing for Child Welfare Practice: Themes, a Cognitive-Affective Model, and Implications from a Qualitative Study." Coleman, Daniel, and Sherrill Clark. Co-published simultaneously in *Journal of Human Behavior in the Social Environment* (The Haworth Social Work Practice Press, an imprint of The Haworth Press, Inc.) Vol. 7, No. 1/2, 2003, pp. 83-96; and: *Charting the Impacts of University-Child Welfare Collaboration* (ed: Katharine Briar-Lawson, and Joan Levy Zlotnik) The Haworth Social Work Practice Press, an imprint of The Haworth Press, Inc., 2003, pp. 83-96. Single or multiple copies of this article are available for a fee from The Haworth Document Delivery Service [1-800-HAWORTH, 9:00 a.m. - 5:00 p.m. (EST). E-mail address: getinfo@haworthpressinc.com].

plications are explored for graduate programs, professors, and supervisors. *[Article copies available for a fee from The Haworth Document Delivery Service: 1-800-HAWORTH. E-mail address: <getinfo@haworthpressinc.com> Website: <http://www.HaworthPress.com> © 2003 by The Haworth Press, Inc. All rights reserved.]*

KEYWORDS. Child welfare, training, developmental perspective

INTRODUCTION

Public child welfare practice is widely recognized to be one of the most challenging areas of social work practice (Bunston, 1997; Dane, 2000). The child welfare worker is faced with some of the most emotional situations that human beings experience: encountering children and families reeling from painful episodes of abuse and neglect, and often faced with parents and children broken apart physically and emotionally as families and as individuals by these events. Simultaneously, the child welfare worker is expected to represent and implement laws and policies while attempting to advocate for their clients in a social service environment with often scarce resources. How do we prepare MSW students to work in this field? What are some unifying themes that help us understand the challenge that faces students, educators, and supervisors?

This paper seeks to provide answers to these questions through the analysis of the results of thirty-seven focus groups conducted over four years with approximately 550 Title IV-E MSW students in California. The focus groups were part of the evaluation efforts of the California Social Work Education Center (CalSWEC) in the fourteen participating graduate schools of social work in California. The themes that emerged in the focus groups pointed to the need to understand child welfare work from a developmental perspective that embraces both cognitive and emotional dimensions. This paper develops a cognitive-affective model that will aid educators to target their teaching and training efforts. This model has important implications for social work educators, child welfare supervisors and administrators and for policy makers with an interest in increasing the quality of child welfare services. This working model should continue to be tested and elaborated through ongoing quantitative and qualitative studies.

Literature Review

There is surprisingly little literature on the emotional needs of social work students. As suggested earlier, it is first important to acknowledge the intense emotional issues confronted by parents, children and workers in child welfare interventions. The retention of child welfare workers was not a primary concern of this study, but it is clearly related to the intensity and complexity of work with clients, and the atmosphere and level of support that an agency provides. Dickinson and Perry (1998), in a large sample quantitative study, found that burnout and "emotional exhaustion" are a concern of workers at all levels in the child welfare system, and was associated with workers leaving child welfare work. Several small sample qualitative studies have also addressed the issue of retention of child welfare workers, identifying the personal and agency qualities that contributed to decisions to stay in child welfare practice (Reagh, 1994; Rycraft, 1994).

The aforementioned studies focused on practitioners who had been in the field for some years. This study gathers data from MSW students who have had a minimum of one field placement in child welfare, as they embark on a two-year commitment to practice in child welfare. What are the challenges, fears and skills that are salient at this beginning stage? Cohen (1994) conducted an exploratory study which indirectly touches on this issue in describing the emotional perspectives of culturally diverse social work students. The author notes that there were concerns expressed about the use of self, amount of self-disclosure, and fear of over-involvement. Countertransference is probably the most frequent framework for discussing students' emotional responses to social work training and education process (see Tosone, 1998, for a literature review). Transference refers to the feelings from other intense relationships that clients project onto practitioners. Countertransference refers to the emotional responses of practitioners to clients, both those derived from the practitioner's own psychology and history, and those evoked by the client's transferences. An example that occurs frequently in child welfare work is the transference of a child placed in foster care onto their worker as a parental figure. The worker's countertransference to this demanding emotional role can range from pleasure and satisfaction, to feeling they must save the child, or anger at the child's biological parents.

Young (1994) wrote about leading a clinical supervision group of child welfare MSW students. One focus that emerged in this group was the need to develop an understanding of transference and countertransference, grounded in the students' own practice experiences. Over the course of a year, students identified ambivalence about the use of authority, feelings of vulnerability in "slowing down" to explore the dynamics of their cases, and dealing with the issues of loss and separation inherent in child protective work. Grossman, Levine-Jordano, and Shearer (1991) recognized the role of emotion for social work trainees and proposed a model for normalizing student's emotional response to field experiences and for integrating an affective component into field supervision.

Bunston (1997) analyzed the emotional impact of child protective work using both transference/countertransference and systems ideas. She writes: "The emotional toll of protective work appears too complex and often too painful to address, often resulting in a high turnover of staff and low professional recognition . . ." (p. 61). The ". . . too complex . . . and painful to address. . ." suggests an emotional push to use simpler cognitive processes. As an adaptive strategy, child welfare workers may be impelled to view children and families more as bureaucratic entities than as complex interactions between stressed family members.

The literature on vicarious traumatization of psychotherapists working with sexually and physically abused clients has relevance to child protective workers as well (Neumann & Gamble, 1995). Vicarious traumatization recognizes the emotional and psychological impact of working day after day with the intimate details of abuse and neglect, and witnessing the traumatic impact on children and families of these events. These impacts may be exacerbated in child welfare workers by having to experience first hand the living situations of their clients, and by having to make weighty decisions in short time frames. Dane (2000) applied the clinical construct of vicarious traumatization to the experience of child welfare workers, and suggested a program to aid workers to use more adaptive coping strategies.

The emotional dimension of child welfare work, then, is in a relationship of mutual influence with the "cognitive set" of the worker. Like the colloquial "mind set," cognitive set is used here to evoke certain assumptions and belief patterns which workers use to interpret information and make decisions. When presented with an overwhelming emotional situation, workers may retreat from emotions and complexity, and fall back onto the unsophisticated application of agency regulations. Decisions are then made on the basis of regulation oriented formulas. While cognitive level may tumble under the pressure of intense emotional situations, more complex and emotionally aware cognitive functioning may allow the integration and management of affect (Goleman, 1995). How, then, do we conceptualize students' cognitive-affective functioning? The measures used in studies of social work students built on previous stage theories of cognitive development (Erwin, 1983; Perry, 1970; Martin et al., 1994). Each of the theorists use slightly different labels for their stages, but all three are working within a tradition and building on each other's work. We will use the work of Martin et al. (1994) to guide our cognitive-affective stages, as this work is the most current empirical research available. Here we will define three stages that summarize these approaches to cognitive development, and emphasize the interrelationship of cognitive level and emotional coping style (see Figure 1).

The absolutist level, the first stage of cognitive development, is characterized by an appeal to authority to define right and wrong and the reliance on rules to guide decision making. At the absolutist level, affect and emotion is relegated to a secondary role to "doing what you have to do." The second stage, relativism, centers on an ability to recognize multiple viewpoints and that one's own perspective is subjective. The relativist, however, is prone to concluding that there is no basis for assessing the relative truthfulness of different accounts of reality. The relativist may value emotion but will not integrate affective responses within a cohesive intellectual framework. This may lead to impulsive actions, "it felt right," or to a paralysis of action in an inability to make difficult value-based decisions. The third stage, critical thinking, incorporates the awareness of complexity in the relativist stage, while recognizing that human beings must select from competing perspectives using value judgements. At this third stage, the authors discuss such ideas as commitment and empathy, and here emotion is integrated into overarching value-based perspectives.

FIGURE 1. Levels of Cognitive-Affective Development

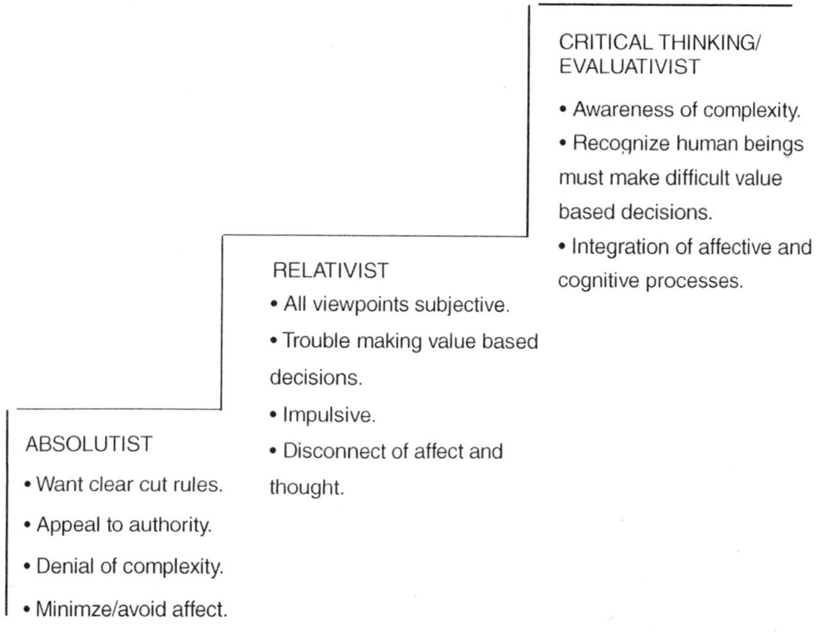

CRITICAL THINKING/
EVALUATIVIST

• Awareness of complexity.

• Recognize human beings
must make difficult value
based decisions.

• Integration of affective and
cognitive processes.

RELATIVIST

• All viewpoints subjective.

• Trouble making value based
decisions.

• Impulsive.

• Disconnect of affect and
thought.

ABSOLUTIST

• Want clear cut rules.

• Appeal to authority.

• Denial of complexity.

• Minimze/avoid affect.

Absolutist workers will make decisions based on formulas found in manuals or passed down by supervisors, and will be unable to weigh complex issues such as effects on children's developmental trajectories, attachment issues, or cultural factors in child rearing practices, to name only a few. Relativist workers, on the other hand, will disavow making difficult discriminations on the basis that there is no way to choose among competing perspectives or choices. Relativist workers will tend to be passive, allowing others to make decisions, or postponing action until mandated interventions are required. Critically thinking workers weigh the complex perspectives involved in a practice situation, consider the ethics and values that underlie different views, and include an assessment of the emotional features (both their own, and others). It is at the critical thinking level that the emotional experience of the worker can be usefully integrated into practice.

In addition to the level of cognitive-affective functioning of the worker, there is the influence of the agency. Studies of policemen, teachers, and social workers identified the individual and institutional push for civil servants to simplify their jobs (Lipsky, 1980; Scott, 1997). This street-level bureaucrat theory argues that workers are impelled to "routinize" their jobs as a defense against the difficult emotions and decisions inherent in their work, and in response to bureaucratic pressures to process a high number of cases (Meyers, Glaser, & McDonald, 1998). These types of bureaucratic pressures encourage absolutist workers, while critically-thinking workers are more likely to resist routinizing their work.

The proposed cognitive-affective model helps to conceptualize the experience of MSW students, and allows an entry point for designing targeted educational interventions. There has been little research on how educational experiences can prepare workers for the complex emotional challenges of practice. In an analogous domain, research in the field of death and dying suggests that education can have beneficial effects in preparing workers to cope with human trauma (Kleespies, 1998, p. 2). Curriculum, class exercises, and supervision interactions that use the developmental cognitive-affective framework are likely to help students better adapt to the challenges of child welfare work. This framework may also be helpful for students and practitioners in other areas of social work practice.

Methods

Student focus groups have been conducted near the end of the 1994-1995, 1995-1996, and 1997-1998 school years in most of the 14 schools of social work in California that are in partnership with CalSWEC. The total number of focus groups conducted, taped and transcribed is thirty-seven. Since this is group level data, exact counts of participants were not collected in two of the three years. In the one year where participants were counted (1996), the average number of participants was 15 (excluding one group that had only 3 participants, and one where no count was conducted). An estimate of total sample size is 550 (37 groups averaging 15 participants each). The groups are conducted in the student's last semester of MSW study, and it is estimated that 75 to 80 percent of the graduating California IV-E students have participated in the focus groups. The focus groups followed a semi-structured format with probes of student views of the specialized child welfare curriculum. Although the emotional challenge of child welfare work was not part of the question protocol, the theme spontaneously emerged in many groups, and was present as a sub-text in most if not all of the groups.

This research was reviewed by the Committee for the Protection of Human Subjects (CPHS) at the University of California, Berkeley, and declared to be in a category exempt from full review. Group participants are assured of confidentiality and of the voluntary nature of their participation. Informed consent was elicited both verbally and in writing.

In this study, a hybrid of traditional read and reread coding and of text searches for certain words was employed (Buston, 1997). The qualitative analysis software package NUD*IST (Qualitative Solutions and Research, 1997) was used both to organize coding and to perform automated keyword searches. All keyword searches were "cleaned" of irrelevant hits, and random checks of comprehensiveness were conducted. Line by line coding serves as a procedural check, insuring that the researcher's thinking stays close to the actual words spoken by the subjects. Themes and coding were reviewed by both authors in an iterative process that led to the development of more abstract ideas, or theory. This method of coding and grouping in categories is the core qualitative analytic technique in common to many specific methods (Denzin and Lincoln, 1994).

As noted, the semi-structured interview format did not directly question emotional and cognitive approaches to field work. The most frequent manifest themes in the groups clustered around a focus on direct practice preparation. As the authors explored these categories of themes, the unifying interpretive structure of the emotional challenge of practice and a range of cognitive-affective responses emerged. These hypotheses were then tested by returning to the transcripts of the groups and seeking examples of these themes, as well as for examples that falsify or contradict the hypothesized interpretive framework. The reader is invited to reflect about the verbatim focus group material presented below and critically appraise the interpretive framework proposed by the authors.

FINDINGS

The most frequent themes of the focus groups centered on direct practice. Paradoxically, students emphasized direct practice as the most frequently mentioned strength of the curriculum as well as the most frequently mentioned weakness. This fact underlines students' preoccupation with being prepared for the challenging situations of practice. The counts of themes found in this study are reported elsewhere (Coleman & Clark, 1998). As the authors explored the student's comments in the focus groups, anxiety and apprehension about the emotional challenge of child welfare work emerged as a theme. Further, it became evident that the students had different styles of handling this challenge that reasonably corresponded to the absolutist, relativist, and critical thinking model of cognitive-affective development. This section uses summaries of student comments and direct quotes to first profile the emotional impact of child welfare, and then illustrate the three stage cognitive-affective hierarchy.

The Emotional Impact

Highly representative of the feelings stirred up by child welfare work is the following statement of a group member about a child who lost a "good placement":

> Eventually, they kicked her out. I cried about that one. Now she will be in another home and things will happen to her all over again. I felt like no one would ever love her. I had thought that this family was her last chance. She had started to make progress, and they were really dedicated to her. Now I feel she will be bounced around in group homes until she is 18.

Another student spoke of the difficulty in knowing what was appropriate affect to feel and show:

> When I had to tell a mom her 12 months were up, she had six more months. Basically, I let her know we were looking at adoption. I had to watch her cry. I'm human. I knew that she hadn't been doing much to reunify with her children. I didn't want to cry in front of her.

Specific to the emotional issues inherent in beginning practice, an older psychotherapist once remarked to one of us (DC) that in the first several years of psychotherapy practice there was a natural terror about one's ability to bear the pain and need for nurturance of a caseload of clients. The different experience of a child welfare job may mitigate some terrors and exacerbate others compared with psychotherapy practice. The issue of caseload and the inherent contradictions of meeting bureaucratic guidelines and providing service to children and families is encapsulated in the following statement:

> What I never heard in class is how you can do anything with 70-80 cases. What did we have in school that taught us how do deal with that as well as help anybody? It really scares people away from certain units. You will lose good workers.

The preceding quotations illustrate that child welfare workers are challenged to work with intense emotional situations under the pressure of high caseloads. No matter the overall cognitive affective level of the worker, child welfare work will be very challenging. However, at more advanced levels of cognitive-affective functioning, the worker is more likely to be able to place the emotion they are experiencing into a meaningful context. In the next section the student's comments will demonstrate how the cognitive-affective levels are manifested in child welfare practice.

Cognitive-Affective Levels

One contributor to the focus groups' emphasis on basic training for child welfare practice is that the anxiety about the challenging role of child welfare practice is handled by becoming preoccupied with the technical aspects of the job. Students feel that if they know all of the specific assessment criteria and laws, then they will be able to handle the large caseload and the complex family issues. This strategy is the absolutist solution–the job is the application of black and white rules to situations. Of course individual agencies, and units within agencies, vary in their work culture including the recognition of the child welfare work as a complex cognitive-affective process. Some work cultures encourage critical thinking workers, where others favor the absolutist approach.

The following student comment reflects the pragmatism of the absolutist cognitive-affective set, and of the sense of urgency to be prepared for practice:

> Forget about the history. My classmates thought I was funny when I said the first day of class that I didn't want to hear about anything that happened before 1980. I need something I can use right now if I go out on the line.

In this next statement, a student is discussing having received classroom instruction on several "theoretical" ways to approach assessment:

> After a while, when you get into the county, things are done, but they are formatted. When you are actually putting it into practice, you don't have time to think about taking a theory and applying it.

The paradox of the absolutist solution to the problem of beginning practice is the question of whether the flawless bureaucratic worker can do sound, ethical social work. Absolutist workers may also be vulnerable to burnout and stress related illnesses because they are avoiding the emotional dimension of practice. While an absolutist worker attempts to apply clear-cut rules, they are forever stymied by a world that is shades of gray.

The MSW social worker is intended to be able to approach the tasks and problems of social work in a more complex and contextualized manner, to understand the need for flexibility and an appreciation for the inherent contradictions and ambiguities of social work practice (Harrison & Atherton, 1990). This goal of MSW education is reflected in the critical thinking stage of the cognitive-affective development schema.

The following comment reflects the student's awareness of complexity, and the relativism of different perspectives on practice situations:

> Self awareness is very important. It is almost impossible to be a good social worker and not be self aware. We run into so many diverse clients we need to be aware of any biases we might have.

Another student discussed the necessity to be able to apply theoretical knowledge to practice situations, and to be able to interpret this knowledge to clients:

> You are dealing with children so you have to have a good understanding of developmental milestones of children. You need to be able to assist the families in identifying these milestones as normal occurrences when the parents may translate them as abnormal or obnoxious.

The following comment exemplifies the critical thinking approach to practice:

> I think personally I did have some struggle in the beginning of my internship because I wanted to do what was correct for the agency. In trying to follow policy, I would sometimes forget about advocacy. Being an intern, I often didn't want to go for it because something else might be jeopardized that might harm my studies or whatever. Coming back and reviewing those things I saw different approaches.

This student felt the push to work from an absolutist framework—"to do what was correct." However, he or she weighed the risks of harming his or her academic progress, and weighed the perspectives of the agency, and of a value of advocating and empowering clients. It is this openness to ambiguity and multiple perspectives that is one goal of graduate social work training. The other is the ability to make value-informed decisions and actions with an awareness that it is based on limited information, and bound by one's own perspective.

A student identified the practice class as catalyzing a change in how he or she thought and felt about child welfare practice:

> The practice class raised my standards from before. Before I did this job I responded like I think. Now I care more. I see more interventions. I have more concern about helping . . .

A theme emerged in the groups of certain classroom techniques that the students credited with helping advance their learning, and their emotional coping with practice. A student contributed the following comment:

> Oral presentations and case presentations. The class being involved in the case. Just hearing experiences from other students not only helped me professionally but helped me to work through my own issues or feelings about frustrations. I had no other way of knowing that other students were going through some of those same experiences. It was very validating and informative.

DISCUSSION

The themes that emerged in the focus groups tell of the emotional challenge of child welfare work, and suggest three distinct cognitive-affective modes of approach. The students' comments themselves also suggested the pathway to facilitating movement to more advanced cognitive-affective levels: the opportunity to talk about case material, to receive support from peers, and to share ideas about how to respond to specific situations. These classroom case discussions also include an emotional component of mutual support, and of suggesting to one another ways of understanding and using the emotions in practice situations. Instructors should be attuned to facilitating these dialogical and supportive processes in the classroom. The exploration of multiple viewpoints in an atmosphere of emotional awareness in the classroom mirrors the intrapersonal process we wish to see students achieve as individuals. Both in the classroom, and within each student, the presence of emotionally aware dialogical processes is a marker that higher level cognitive-affective functioning is taking place.

To model and begin these processes, faculty should illustrate theoretical material with case examples or other connections to the day to day practice of child welfare. Students liked courses which used actual cases to explore the content areas of the course. This needn't be isolated to practice courses or field seminars. Case material can be used to illustrate policy dilemmas, principles of child development, and theories of treatment. Faculty could improve their credibility, and gain material for integrating course material with the practice world, through spending some time in child welfare agencies and observing child welfare workers in action. The use of case material can allow students to experience the complexities and ambiguities of practice without the weighty pressures of real life practice. Faculty who have experienced front-line practice can model a dialogical and emotionally self-aware stance to practice, to help students to advance in their capacity to tolerate the conflicting feelings and the inherent ambiguity of direct practice.

Schools and individual instructors may wish to examine the issue of the prevailing level of cognitive-affective development of students, and to tailor learning experiences to work toward the goal of a more advanced and flexible cognitive-affective process. Seminar classes where an atmosphere of trust and acceptance has been established may permit students to discuss the complex web of emotions and thoughts involved in beginning practice. This will facilitate support from the instructor and other students, allowing a loosening of the emotional pressure on the student. Students showed an appreciation for opportunities to talk honestly with one another about practice. Dane's (2000) small focus group study with child welfare workers also suggested a similar group model for child welfare workers to develop their understanding and coping skills with emotional stress. Perhaps the emotional component should be explicitly included in curricula and syllabi to remind all participants to attend to this important area, and to endorse classroom time spent on the students' emotional responses.

Programs, instructors and supervisors who are mindful of both the affective and the cognitive dimensions of the training and education process seem more likely to meet the needs of their students. If the student's fears about practice are not addressed, they are more likely to use a absolutist approach in their work. Alternately, we feel that students who use critical thinking are more able to manage the emotional demands of child welfare work. If schools of social work produce absolutist child welfare workers, the aims of professionalization are defeated. Students have to be encouraged to see beyond the routine application of codes and regulations: at stake is not only the lives of children and families, but also their own mental health and the sustainability of practicing as a child welfare worker.

This study worked from the verbatim statements of the students themselves. Future research could use quantitative methods and random sampling to test the ideas emergent in this study. Educators could test cognitive-affective functioning of students using a measure of cognitive level (Martin et al., 1994), or emotional intelligence (Schutte et al., 1998). Testing early in a course would allow assessment of how students at different levels respond to educational techniques. Testing later in a course could allow an assessment of effectiveness of the overall curriculum, or of specific modules. This type of correlational study is highly feasible, as it only requires completing short paper and pencil inventories.

Although more complex and costly, the true frontier in research on child welfare education is studies that examine effects on client outcomes. Possible outcome measures vary from the average duration of a worker's caseload in foster care, to client ratings of satisfaction with a worker, or, ultimately, measures of developmental outcomes of clients.

WORKS CITED

Bunston, Wendy. (1997). Encouraging therapeutic reflection in child and adolescent protective services. *Australian & New Zealand Journal of Family Therapy*, *18*(2), 61-69.

Buston, K. (1997). NUD*IST in action: its use and its usefulness in a study of chronic illness in young people. *Sociological Research Online*, *2*(3). <http://www.socresonline. org.uk/socresonline/2/3/6.html>.

Cohen, C. (1994). What culturally diverse students say about emotion: an exploratory study. *Journal of Multicultural Social Work*, *3*(1), 113-124.

Coleman, D., Clark, S. J. (1998). *The Student Focus Groups: IV-E Students Speak Out on the Classroom Curriculum*. Report to the Board of the California Social Work Education Center. October 2, 1998.

Dane, B. (2000). Child welfare workers: an innovative approach for interacting with secondary trauma. *Journal of Social Work Education*, *36*(1), 27-38.

Denzin, N. K., Lincoln, Y. S. (1994). Entering the field of qualitative research. In *Handbook of qualitative research*, (N.K. Denzin, Y.S Lincoln, eds.) Thousand Oaks, CA: Sage Publications.

Dickinson, N., Perry, R. (1998). *Do MSW graduates stay in public child welfare? Factors influencing the burnout and retention rates of specially educated child welfare workers*. Paper presented at the conference of the National Association for Welfare Research and Statistics, Chicago IL, August 4, 1998.

Erwin, T. D. (1983). The scale of intellectual development: measuring Perry's scheme. *Journal of College Student Personnel*, *24*, 6-12.

Goleman, D. (1995). *Emotional intelligence*. New York, NY : Bantam.

Grossman, B., Levine-Jordano, N., Shearer, P. (1991). Working with students' emotional reactions in the field: An educational framework. In Schneck, D., Grossman, B., Glassman, U. (Eds.). *Field Education in Social Work: Contemporary Issues and Trends.* Dubuque, IA: Kendall/Hunt.

Harrison, D.W., Kwong K., Cheong, K.J. (1989). Undergraduate education and cognitive development of MSW students: a follow-up to Specht, Britt, and Frost. *Social Research and Abstracts, 25*(2), 15-19.

Harrison, D. W., Atherton, C. R. (1990). Cognitive development and the "One Foundation" controversy. *Journal of Social Work Education, 26*(1), 87-95.

Kleespies, P. (1998). Introduction. In, P. Kleespies (Ed.), *Emergencies in mental health practice: evaluation and management.* New York, NY: Guilford Press.

Lipsky, M. (1980). *Street-level bureaucracy: dilemmas of the individual in public services.* New York, NY: Russell Sage Foundation.

Martin, J.E., Silva, D.G., Newman, J.H., Thayer, J.F. (1994). An investigation into the structure of epistemological style. *Personality & Individual Differences, 16* (4), 617-629.

Meyers, M. K., Glaser, B., Mac Donald, K. (1998). On the front lines of welfare delivery: are workers implementing policy reforms? *Journal of Policy Analysis & Management, 17*(1), 1-22.

Neumann, D. A., Gamble, S. J. (1995). Issues in the professional development of psychotherapists: Countertransference and vicarious traumatization in the new trauma therapist. *Psychotherapy, 32*(2), 341-347.

Perry, W. G. (1970). *Forms of intellectual and ethical development in the college years.* New York, NY: Holt, Rinehart and Winston.

Qualitative Solutions and Research. (1997). *QSR NUD*IST 4.0.* Melbourne: QSR.

Schutte, N. S., Malouff, J. M., Hall, L. E., Haggerty, D.J., & others. (1998). Development and validation of a measure of emotional intelligence. *Personality & Individual Differences, 25*(2), 167-177.

Scott, Patrick G. (1997). Assessing determinants of bureaucratic discretion: an experiment in street-level decision making. *Journal of Public Administration Research and Theory, 7*(1).

Tosone, C. (1998). Countertransference and clinical social work supervision: Contributions and considerations. *Clinical Supervisor, 16*(2), 17-32.

Young, T. M. (1994). Collaboration of a public child welfare agency and a school of social work: a clinical group supervision project. *Child Welfare, 73*(6), 659-671.

Preparing Social Work Students for Interdisciplinary Practice: Learnings from a Curriculum Development Project

Bart Grossman

Kathleen McCormick

SUMMARY. This article reports findings of an MSW interdisciplinary practice curriculum experiment. A diverse group of students at ten schools of social work were provided with specialized fieldwork and training. The agencies represented a broad array of services, fields of practice client populations and professional disciplines. Students encountered frequent interdisciplinary disputes and often found social workers coordinating interdisciplinary teams, a role upon which social work curricula rarely focus. This specialized experience seems to have

Bart Grossman, PhD, MSW, is Adjunct Profesor and Director of Fieldwork at the University of California at Berkeley, School of Social Welfare. He was Founding Director of the California Social Work Education Center and has written extensively on field education and child welfare education in social work.

Kathleen McCormick, MSW, is a former PhD candidate at the University of California at Berkeley, School of Social Welfare. She is a social worker in San Francisco Bay Area with a background in substance abuse and medical social services

This research was supported by the California Social Work Education Center, University of California at Berkeley and by a grant from the Administration for Children and Families, Department of Health and Human Services.

[Haworth co-indexing entry note]: "Preparing Social Work Students for Interdisciplinary Practice: Learning from a Curriculum Development Project." Grossman, Bart, and Kathleen McCormick. Co-published simultaneously in *Journal of Human Behavior in the Social Environment* (The Haworth Social Work Practice Press, an imprint of The Haworth Press, Inc.) Vol. 7, No. 1/2, 2003, pp. 97-113; and: *Charting the Impacts of University-Child Welfare Collaboration* (ed: Katharine Briar-Lawson, and Joan Levy Zlotnik) The Haworth Social Work Practice Press, an imprint of The Haworth Press, Inc., 2003, pp. 97-113. Single or multiple copies of this article are available for a fee from The Haworth Document Delivery Service [1-800-HAWORTH, 9:00 a.m. - 5:00 p.m. (EST). E-mail address: getinfo@haworthpressinc.com].

not only enriched students' preparation for interdisciplinary work, but also deepened their understanding of social work as a unique discipline. *[Article copies available for a fee from The Haworth Document Delivery Service: 1-800-HAWORTH. E-mail address: <getinfo@haworthpressinc.com> Website: <http://www.HaworthPress.com> © 2003 by The Haworth Press, Inc. All rights reserved.]*

KEYWORDS. Interdisciplinary practice, curriculum development, teams, multidisciplinary

INTRODUCTION

This article reports findings of an MSW interdisciplinary practice curriculum experiment. A diverse group of students at ten school of social work in California were provided with specialized fieldwork and training. Their experiences and learnings were documented to see what effect the specialized training would have on their level of preparation for and identification with professional social work.

An interest in interdisciplinary preparation for the helping professions emerged in the 1980s in response to a social service system increasingly seen as fractured and ineffective (Lawson and Hooper-Briar, 1994A). The professional literature had began to feature new coordinated models of service delivery (Brill, 1976; Anderson and Shaefer, 1979; Faller, 1981; Barker, 1989; Baglow, 1990). However, professional education showed little response to these efforts at first. In fact, Lawson and Hooper-Briar (1994) suggest that education for the helping professions within higher education is, "among the primary producers of categorical thinking and policies" (p. 13). The reasons for this situation include the pressures of tenure, the expansiveness of accreditation requirements, and the competitiveness of professional schools in a time of shrinking educational resources.

Institutions of higher education are often cited as among the most conservative of institutions; social service agencies and their policies are among the most mercurial. Support for professional education in Universities depends highly on governmental financing. Beginning in the 1980s, such funding began to have interprofessional "strings attached." As a result, many innovative, interprofessional education efforts have been launched.

Jivanjee et al. (1995), describe 51 such programs, 26 agency training efforts, and 25 university professional education programs, including the one described in this paper. Most had some multidisciplinary course planning (88%)

and team teaching (92%), and nineteen of the university programs involved common fieldwork among the disciplines. Interestingly, only four of the University projects and none of the agency programs had a written definition of "interprofessional."

When we set out to prepare professionals to lead and serve in interdisciplinary/interprofessional delivery systems, we immediately encounter a serious difficulty. It seems there is little clarity about what these terms mean. Hooper-Briar and Lawson (1994) identify five kinds of service integration B client-centered, provider-centered, program-centered, organization-centered and policy-centered. Each implies different kinds and degrees of collaboration among disciplines.

Similarly, the authors have noted a range of practices that are referred to under the rubric of interdisciplinary collaboration. These include:

- *Cross-system communication*–encouraging collaboration among professionals in separate delivery systems who are sometimes from different educational backgrounds but just as often have the same professional degrees. For example, a strong antipathy has existed for years between social workers in child welfare and in mental health who frequently serve the same clients,
- *Diffusion of knowledge*–educating one professional field in knowledge traditionally reserved to another (e.g., teaching social workers about human biology and physicians about interpersonal skills),
- *Service merger*–placing professionals formally associated with separate agencies into a reconstituted delivery system (e.g., integrating child mental health, child welfare and developmental disabilities into a single children's service agency),
- *Interprofessional sensitivity training*–teaching professionals or pre-professional students to understand each other and work together more effectively through common course work, fieldwork, or conferences and workshops, and
- *Creating new professions*–developing educational programs and departments that cut across old disciplinary distinctions such as degrees in human services, child welfare, aging and drug addiction.

In professional and vocational education it is more the norm than an exception for practice in the field, to have advanced beyond the current state of knowledge and theory. Faculty must frequently prepare students for a reality that is unclear and unstable. The continuing centrality of field experience within social work education has allowed it to move beyond the scope of existing curriculum and formulate education "on the fly." As Schneck (1990) describes this process:

> Knowledge can inform practice, but practice can also reform knowledge. We may, at times, have a better configuration of practice, construed artfully and intuitively in fieldwork than would be had by the integration of existing, perhaps even outmoded, ideas and methods. On that occasion, our obligation would be to "disintegrate" the configuration, articulate the policy, method, and content issues back to the classroom and researchers. (p. 56)

The report that follows describes a project that sought to learn about how to educate students for interdisciplinary practice by placing them in interdisciplinary fieldwork, offering them the best information available at the time and learning from their experience.

THE CALSWEC INTERDISCIPLINARY PROGRAM

In 1991, the California Social Work Education Center (CalSWEC) was awarded a five-year Interdisciplinary Child Welfare Grant by the Children's Bureau of the Administration on Children and Families (Department of Health and Social Services). It was the largest of eleven such grants throughout the United States. At that time CalSWEC was a newly formed coalition of ten schools of social work and 58 county departments of social services with administrative funding from the Ford Foundation. It had the mission of expanding and enhancing MSW child welfare training in California. Work was underway to develop standard curriculum competencies and to secure funding for MSW educational stipends.

Preparation for interdisciplinary practice was not an explicit mission of CalSWEC, since its founders were concerned with what they believed to be a more pressing and basic concern: getting social workers prepared for and committed to work in public child welfare at a time when the profession seemed to be abandoning this field. It is also fair to say that the RFP for this grant offered little guidance about how the "interdisciplinary" focus should be reflected.

As the project emerged, the Interdisciplinary Training Program was designed to accelerate development of the central CalSWEC effort while allowing exploration of specialized education for interdisciplinary practice. The term "interdisciplinary" was understood in two ways:

- as a range of knowledge from a wide variety of disciplines (social work, law, mental health, medicine and public health, and management and public administration) required for effective professional social work practice in child welfare (*Diffusion of Knowledge*) and,

- as a set of skills needed by social workers to effectively communicate with and link other professionals involved in serving child welfare clients (*Interprofessional Sensitivity*).

While child welfare curriculum content was being upgraded in all of the participating schools, there was little specific consideration of preparation for work with other professions and fields. The Interdisciplinary Training Program was, therefore, infused with interdisciplinary content and experiences in the second sense mentioned above.

The Program provided an educational stipend of $8,000 to a second-year student at each of the MSW programs in the state of California. The program was restricted to second-year students because first year fieldwork is rather truncated at several of the schools. It was considered important that the students be socialized as social workers in the field prior to participation in the interdisciplinary experience. In addition, these students:

- Completed second-year fieldwork in specialized innovative child welfare settings, either public or non-profit, that featured work with multidisciplinary teams,
- Attended a start-up workshop on interdisciplinary child welfare
- practice and teamwork,
- Attended a week-long interdisciplinary child welfare workshop at California State University at San Diego, and
- Completed special writing assignments on interdisciplinary work.

The workshops offered a foundation in interdisciplinary and child welfare content based on the experience of an existing program at San Diego State University. However, it was felt faculty and agencies could best develop effective interdisciplinary curriculum content collaboratively by following students engaged in interdisciplinary fieldwork. Each school selected a setting that involved, at a minimum, three human services professions in addition to social work. While the settings could be under the auspices of public agencies, they were not traditional service delivery models, but rather community-based or inter-system collaboratives seeking to serve clients holistically rather than categorically.

DATA COLLECTION AND PROCESSING

The Interdisciplinary Training Program was run in 1992-93 and 1993-94. Basic reaction data were collected at the end of each year. However, student data collected at the end of a program often suffer from a high level of particularism and a lack of perspective. Therefore, the project staff planned to interview all the participants at least six months after graduation.

A doctoral research assistant with a strong interdisciplinary practice background played a central role in the data collection process. An interview protocol (appended), was developed by the project director and research assistant. About half of the items requested demographic and descriptive information. The remaining items probed the students' perceptions of interdisciplinary practice in their field settings, their evaluation of the strengths and weaknesses of various facets of their education and their suggestions for future interdisciplinary education.

Eighteen of the 20 student participants were successfully surveyed in 1995-96, via a telephone interview lasting about sixty minutes. All of the phone interviews were conducted by the research assistant. The findings of these surveys are the basis of this report. Some collateral information from phone interviews field instructors will also be reported.

The interview findings were transcribed and entered into the NUD.IST qualitative analysis computer program (Richards, T.J., and Richards, L. (1991). A set of categories was developed inductively from the NUD.IST entries. Initially the project director and the research assistant independently developed categories. The two sets of categories were then combined to achieve a unified set. The categories and numbers of responses are described below. The sample size was judged to preclude meaningful use of statistical procedures. The numbers can only offer a general indication of the pervasiveness of particular experiences and perceptions that may be tested in future investigations. Examples of comments and direct quotations are utilized where possible to help specify participants' meanings.

Given the small size and the uniqueness of settings and experiences these findings cannot offer overarching conclusions about the nature and consequences of interdisciplinary training in social work However, they may provide insights into student learning and the unique challenges and opportunities available in interdisciplinary venues that will be of use to other programs. It is also hoped that they will be a contribution to a field in which writing has thus far been largely speculative.

FINDINGS

Student Demographics

Items one through five dealt with basic identifying information about the students. Some suggestive comparisons can be made with data on the overall population of MSW students in California schools conducted annually by CalSWEC. Of note in this regard is the fact that the mean age of project students was 33, slightly higher than the mean age of 31 for California students in 1993 (n = 917). Also there were substantially more participants of color in the interdisciplinary program than the proportion in the overall student population (see Table 1).

Students in the program had an average of two years of practice experience. While students in the CalSWEC study report more experience (about 30 months), the items in the two surveys were not comparable, as the interdisciplinary survey item explicitly included volunteer experience. Conversations with several California admissions officers, however, suggest that two years of prior experience in social work is a "normal" rate. The program group was thus somewhat older, of comparable experience and more racially diverse than the overall MSW student population in the state in 1993.

Placement Descriptions

The next section of the protocol focused on the student field placement. Students were asked about the type of settings in which they had been placed. Because several agencies were ranked in more than one category, the agency topologies summed to more than 18 (Table 2). Seven of the 18, the largest group, were described as social services/child welfare. Five were children's services, five client advocacy, four mental health and three were described as generic multidisciplinary public agencies. While none of the placements were identified as primarily schools, six included direct responsibility for school-based services. This array fairly reflects the fields in which multidisciplinary innovation has been taking place.

TABLE 1. Percentages of Participants of Color versus Total Student Population in California in 1993.

	Program group	Overall**
African American	20% (4)	13%
American Indian	5% (1)	2%
Asian American	0% (0)	6%
Caucasian	40% (8)	59%
Chicano/Latino	35% (7)	16%

* Comparison based on a survey of all entering students in California, CalSWEC 1993, (n= 917).
** Approximately 4% identified as other or unknown.

TABLE 2. Services Offered

Case Management	4
Crisis Intervention	3
Counseling–Individual	10
Counseling–Group	6
Counseling–Family	7
Therapy	3
I and R	4
Recreation	1
Advocacy	2
Outreach	2
Parent Education	2
School Social Work	1
Educational Programs	3
Health	3
Substance Abuse	1
Consultation	1

TABLE 3. Main Purpose of Placements

Mental Health	5
Family Support/Preservation	3
Other Child Welfare (CPS, Foster Care)	3
School Social Work	2
Health Service	2
Case Management	1
Service Integration	5

As for auspices, half of the placements were in private nonprofit settings, seven were purely public agencies and two were formal public/private partnerships (Table 3). When asked about the types of services of not surprisingly, the most frequent response regarding the main purpose of the setting was mental health.

However, five students felt that their setting had a coequal main purpose of service integration. It is surprising, given the frequent mention of poverty and material need, that none of the students indicated that provision of material resources was a significant purpose of their placement setting.

TABLE 4. Primary Role of Social Work in the Agency

Interdisciplinary Coordination	10
Case Management	6
Family Intervention	3
Generalist Social Work	3
I and R	3
Administration	3
Counseling/Therapy	3
Advocacy	2
Primary Caregiver	2
Represent Social Work Point of View	2
Supervision	1

The client groups served by students were primarily inner-city minorities. Latinos and African Americans were far more frequently mentioned than Caucasians. Young mothers and children were each mentioned as target groups by seven of the 18 respondents, but no other specific age groups were identified. The sorts of problems mentioned reflect the typical situation surrounding poor inner-city families served by the child welfare system, including abuse and neglect, poverty and material needs, child behavior problems, school performance issues, substance abuse and mental health issues.

Interdisciplinary Experience

A series of questions was devoted to the students' impressions of the nature of interdisciplinary work in their settings. Two types of models were identified. The first involved various disciplines collaborating through a formal coordinating agency. The alternative model was a multidisciplinary agency in which the various disciplines were directly employed. Eleven agencies fit the first description while four fit the second type. Three settings were described as possessing the characteristics of both types. Students were asked about the "primary" role social work played in their interdisciplinary setting. Thirteen different primary social work roles were mentioned, most by only a few students (see Table 4).

However, 10 students found that social workers were principally responsible for interdisciplinary coordination in the agency. This is a striking finding, given that few MSW programs focus heavily on preparation for this role.

Students reported dealing regularly with about 10 different disciplines in addition to social workers (Table 5). The most common were identified as

TABLE 5. Disciplines Mentioned

Teachers	17
Paraprofessionals	17
Marriage Family and Child Counselors	15
Mental Health Workers	15
Police	13
Nurses	12
Probation Officers	10
Psychologists	8
Doctors	7
Lawyers	4
Ministers	1
Others–Parents, Foster parents, School Administrators, Dentists	4

teachers,paraprofessionals, marriage family and child counselors and mental health workers. Four of the 18 students found that there were few or no problems between the disciplines. Problems cited with some frequency included interdisciplinary disagreements, inadequate communication, lack of knowledge of the other's perspective and disrespect.

When asked which disciplines they found most difficult to work with, eight students mentioned teachers. The primary complaints were that teachers were "not culturally sensitive" (5), "labeled students" (3), and were "callous" (1). Three students reported difficulty with psychologists citing, in each case, "cultural insensitivity." No other disciplines were mentioned more than once or twice as problematic.

Only two mechanisms were identified by more than one or two students as means of resolving disputes; group discussion and attempts made by the students or their supervisors to educate others about the social work role. Five of the students reported that there were no means available in the agency for settling such disputes.

CURRICULUM AND LEARNING

Interdisciplinary Content

The remainder of the questions concerned the educational program each student experienced and suggestions for improved MSW interdisciplinary education. It is especially gratifying in a program with an interdisciplinary focus that all students reported they were well oriented to the role of each discipline. Interestingly though, the mechanisms by which they became oriented varied quite a bit. Six students reported they acquired this information in the special training programs, four in supervision (although eight of the supervisors report having covered the subject), three each from team meetings and personal contact and two from prior experience.

Students were asked where in their prior social work education they had acquired knowledge for interdisciplinary practice. Fourteen students reported they had some, though limited, exposure. The place of this material in the curriculum was highly unpredictable. No more than two students identified any particular class. The courses mentioned included child welfare, group work, community organization, policy, school social work and multicultural practice.

Faculty confirmed that there was little or no such content in most classes but expected that students had exposure in fieldwork. However, no student cited prior fieldwork as relevant. Most students did report that their supervisor in the special fieldwork had helped them develop skills of interdisciplinary practice. Thirteen cited the supervisory process as most helpful, mentioning such qualities as support ("encouraged me in areas where I felt less secure"), availability, follow-through ("things I felt were missing the instructor made happen") and flexibility ("allowed me to do things that may have been inefficient but let me learn on my own").

When asked about what experiences might have helped them better understand other professions, most students requested more interdisciplinary experience and training. Ten students felt that there should be specific interdisciplinary courses in the MSW curriculum. Their comments reflected a desire for more course work in other disciplines (. . . "too much emphasis on social work alone"), more information on the approaches and goals of other professions, and more opportunity to be taught by other professionals.

Field Instructors and Liaisons

It appeared from student and field instructor comments that the instructors were aware of the special nature of the placement and were particularly active with these students. There were a few mildly stated complaints (for example, seven students felt the need for more time from their field instructors). Students were able to cite specific teachings provided and actions taken by field instructors including: "how to set limits re: issues that might come up between disciplines," "how to approach other disciplines," "ways to mediate between physicians, nurses and teens," "including me in all planning meetings," "telling me who to involve in a case."

Students' comments on their experiences with field liaison faculty tell a different story. Eight students felt they had gotten little or nothing from their field liaison. While five mention that the liaison was helpful in the placement process, in only two cases did the comments suggest that the field liaison played an active role once the placement began. The eight students who commented seemed to see the role of liaison as limited to problem solving, ("I did not need to go to her, but I felt I could have"). Four students who had specific complaints saw the liaison as having failed to deal with a problem, (". . . did not ensure the quality of supervision," "did not follow up on the student's experience"). Only two students reported wanting more contact with the field liaison. Two indicated that the liaison should do a better job linking the field and curriculum, ("needs to key into the models used in the settings and discover how it fits with their (theoretical) model.)"

When asked about the value the program had for them, six students particularly cited the opportunities for interdisciplinary contact and learning:

> . . . destroyed my stereotypes about psychologists.

> Especially helpful to exchange points of view with lawyers; got insight into lawyers' motivation to win a case despite the possible negative effects on the family.

> I feel this is the beginning of something powerful happening in CPS in terms of getting all the disciplines together to find common goals for families.

Additionally, six students mentioned the San Diego Interdisciplinary Child Welfare Conference as having been useful. Twelve participants commented that the program had proven helpful in preparing them for their current position:

> Helped in my work with families and underage clients and in working with the legal system.

> I let other disciplines know when they are stepping over into my role as a social worker.

> It made it less intimidating to work with other disciplines. I learned how to understand their point of view. . . . And process this point of view before responding.

> The program made me more effective and sophisticated in seeking out people in other professions who have similar ideas and building on this commonality to secure their assistance.

DISCUSSION

Clearly the interdisciplinary program was considered a valuable experience by most participants. These former students seem to draw on the experience, and their comments reflect a sense of comfort in interdisciplinary situations. Structured interdisciplinary experiences seem not to have undermined their sense of a distinct social work identity. They articulate social work roles and perspectives in a way that strikes one as more nuanced and differentiated than the average graduate. Perhaps in some way training in interaction with other professionals served to heighten their understanding of and identification with social work.

It is not possible to know whether the prior year of traditional social work placement is important to this outcome. However, it may be that interdisciplinary experience should be a part of social work education not only to increase cross disciplinary skill, but because it can, under some conditions, strengthen social work identification.

The agencies in which these students were placed were primarily linked to child welfare and schools at a time when the benefits of school-linked services were being widely touted. The clients were mostly poor and minority "at risk" children and families. Yet the most common services, indeed the most common purpose of the agency, were identified as mental health related.

While counseling skills may be directly relevant, how is it that there is so little acknowledgment of material need? Why is there not more discussion of concrete services, job-finding, housing, child-care and the like? While an emphasis on integration of disciplines is important, it does not appear that most students experienced a true holistic, integrated service approach in which both material and emotional needs were addressed.

For social work, psychology and other counseling professions, primary attention to the intrapsychic and interpersonal has been an important key to professional status. Yet, interdisciplinary services will be no more effective than traditional services if they fail to address the full range of human needs. Certainly social workers will continue to play a central role in the provision of clinical services. However, this need not be its only path to professional respectability.

An alternative to the counseling role for social work emerges in this study that of interdisciplinary team leadership. The skills that are central to this role, however, have been in decline in social work education in recent years. Group work, problem-solving, conflict resolution, program development and organizational analysis will, if these students' experience is a measure, need to be reinvigorated. While these skill areas are not, perhaps, as recognized as they once were in social work, they are even less frequently considered in the other professions.

There may be a window of opportunity for social work to claim a new centrality based on skills of leadership and coordination. Taking advantage of this opportunity, however, will necessitate significant changes in the content of practice courses. Individual work has long dominated counseling and, therefore, most practice courses. However, group work is the core method of team leadership. Group work in most generic methods curricula is like the chicken in the soup. It's on the label, but there is not much in the can.

Preparation for interdisciplinary roles will also be a serious challenge in fieldwork. It is far easier to organize placement around treatment cases than leadership tasks, but the path of least resistance in this situation can only reinforce the status quo.

This project gives us some insight into the dynamics of interdisciplinary conflict. Clearly most of these settings had not considered the need for conflict resolution mechanisms, perhaps because professionals tend to assume that any difference can be resolved if there is good will. However, not all interdisciplinary conflicts are based on misunderstanding and not all conflicts can be solved by better communication.

Social work and teaching are both relatively low status, "front line" professions. It is not unusual for human beings to fight as hard to avoid last place as they do to achieve first place. Teachers and social workers are socialized to see their professional perspective as a moral imperative. The troubled student in the classroom may be both an oppressed victim of a teacher's insensitivity and an impediment to other students' learning who needs to be removed from the class.

We will need to teach students to listen well, analyze carefully, be persuasive and fight fairly and effectively when necessary.

It is important to understand that professional differences are not the source of every dispute. The social work students in this program were frequently more like the clients in class, race and background than were the other professionals. In such instances the social worker may feel a special responsibility to advocate for the client. Interdisciplinary teams need leaders with the sophistication and group skills to help members recognize and appropriately manage race, class and gender dynamics.

The students tell us that preparing for interdisciplinary practice requires specialized content. Interestingly, preparation also benefits from the oldest teaching approach of all, good attentive field instruction that balances support and challenge. The field instructors in this project were thoughtful, devoted and perhaps somewhat energized by the knowledge that they were offering "special" training. How can we impart this energy to all field instructors? The students were content with little direct contact with field liaisons. That may be as it should. Perhaps liaisons should focus their energy on nurturing, supporting and developing field instructors as the front line educators they must be.

The participants in the interdisciplinary training program have shown us that preparing social workers to serve in the new world of collaboration and service integration will be challenging. This challenge can offer social work education an opportunity to reintegrate unique knowledge and skills, claim a central role in the future, and strengthen the identity of the profession in a way that may also improve outcomes for our clients.

REFERENCES

Anderson, L.M., and Shafer, G. (1979). The character disordered family: a community treatment model for family sexual abuse. *American Journal of Orthopsychiatry*, 49(3), 436-445.

Baglow, L.J. (1990). A multidimensional model for the treatment of child abuse: A framework for cooperation. *Child Abuse and Neglect*, 14, 387-395.

Barker, N.C., ed. (1989). *Child abuse and neglect: An interdisciplinary method of treatment.* Dubuque, Iowa: Kendall-Hunt.

Briar, K., Hansen. V., and Harris, N. (1993). *New partnerships.* Miami: Florida International University.

Brill, N.I., (1976). San Jose, CA: J.B. Lippincott. *Teamwork: Working together in human services.*

Faller, K.C., ed. (1981). *Social work with abused and neglected children: A manual for interdisciplinary practice.* New York: Free Press.

Gardner, Sid. (1993). The ethics of collaboration. *Georgia Academy Journal,* I(1), 2-4.

Hooper-Briar, K., and Lawson, H. (1994). *Serving children, youth and families through interprofessional collaboration and service integration: a framework for action.* Oxford, Ohio: The Danforth Foundation and the Institute for Educational Renewal at Miami University.

Jivanjee, P.R., Moore, K.R., Schultze, K.H., and Fiesen, B.J. (1995). *Interprofessional education for family-centered services: a survey of interprofessional/interdisciplinary training programs.* Portland, Oregon: Portland State University, Research and Training Center on Family Support and Children's Mental Health.

Lawson, H., and Hooper-Briar, K. (1994). *Expanding partnerships: involving colleges and universities in interprofessional education and service integration.* Oxford, Ohio: The Danforth Foundation and the Institute for Educational Renewal at Miami University.

Patti, R.J., and Einbinder, S.D. (1997). *Organizational factors associated with collaborative service arrangements.* Berkeley, CA: California Social Work Education Center.

Richards, T.J., and Richards, L. (1991). The NUD.IST qualitative data analysis system. *Qualitative Sociology.* 14(4), 307-324

Schneck, D., Grossman, B., and Glassman, R. (1990). *Field education in social work practice: contemporary issues and trends.* Dubuque, Iowa: Kendall/Hunt.

APPENDIX I–Interdisciplinary Survey Protocol

How old were you at the time of your placement?

How many years of experience (direct or indirect service) had you had when you started your MSW program?

Where did you go to school?

Who was your field liaison from the school?

Where were you placed?

Who was your field instructor at your placement?

What type of an agency were you working in?

Social services/welfare	Law Enforcement
CBO	DA rep.
Mental Health	Probation
Substance Abuse	School
Public Health	Other

Client Advocate Group (please specify)

Public agency composed of various disciplines

Was it a public or private agency?

public   private

What do you consider to be the main purpose of the agency?

What services were provided?

Where and how were services delivered?

Who were the most common clients that you worked with?

What were the most common problems that these clients presented with in your experiences?

What was the interdisciplinary context in which you were placed?

Different disciplines from various agencies working together under the auspices of a coordinating agency___

Different disciplines from within the agency working together___

Other _____

What disciplines did you deal with on a regular basis?

nurses	law enforcement
educators	MFCC's
paraprofessionals	BSW's
MSW's	mental health workers
psychologists	probation officers
lawyers	other

What did you perceive to be the role of a social worker in this interdisciplinary context?

Do you feel that you were oriented to the role each discipline was expected to play in the interdisciplinary process?

>   yes   no

How was this accomplished?

Now I'm going to ask you some questions regarding interdisciplinary communication.

What kind of problems in communication between disciplines did you notice?

How were interdisciplinary problems resolved? How were they not resolved?

Specific to the disciplines that you worked with, which disciplines were more difficult to work with?

What kind of educational experiences would have assisted you in working with these disciplines?

What educational experiences in your MSW program prepared you for working in this setting?

What aspects of the curriculum could be improved to better assist you in working in this setting?

What assistance did your field instructor/supervisor provide in order for you to work more effectively in this setting?

What were the three most important things you learned from him or her?

What were three things you feel that you should have learned from him or her but didn't?

What assistance did your field liaison provide in order for you to work more effectively in this setting, namely

What were the three most important things that you learned from him or her?

What were the three things that you feel that you should have learned but didn't?

Describe your experiences in being involved in the state-wide MSW interdisciplinary stipend program.

General impressions YY.

Moving Toward Collaboration: Using Funding Streams to Advance Partnerships in Child Welfare Practice

Richard Phillips
Patty Gregory
Mardell Nelson

SUMMARY. Traditionally, organizations serving children and families have focused service delivery by available funding stream criteria. Federal funding streams supported fragmented services by tightly channel-

---

Richard Phillips, PhD, is currently Director of Research and Evaluation for the Idaho Child Welfare Center. Dr. Phillips is a faculty member of the Department of Education, Eastern Washington University, with a joint appointment in the School of Social Work. He has a background in educational administration and teaching, and specializes in evaluation of programs that combine systems to provide social services to children who are not finding success in the public schools.

Patty Gregory, MSW, is the Director for the Idaho Child Welfare Research & Training Center and is on faculty at Eastern Washington University, School of Social Work. She has background working in child protection, children's mental health, foster care and adoption. She teaches in the areas of direct practice, family therapy and field education.

Mardell Nelson, MSW, is currently Program Specialist for the Idaho Department of Health and Welfare, Division of Family and Community Services. She is the Title IV-E contract monitor for Idaho's partnership with Eastern Washington University and has a background in child welfare and social work field education. She specializes in social service program planning, training, mediation and community development.

[Haworth co-indexing entry note]: "Moving Toward Collaboration: Using Funding Streams to Advance Partnerships in Child Welfare Practice." Phillips, Richard, Patty Gregory, and Mardell Nelson. Co-published simultaneously in *Journal of Human Behavior in the Social Environment* (The Haworth Social Work Practice Press, an imprint of The Haworth Press, Inc.) Vol. 7, No. 1/2, 2003, pp. 115-133; and: *Charting the Impacts of University-Child Welfare Collaboration* (ed: Katharine Briar-Lawson, and Joan Levy Zlotnik) The Haworth Social Work Practice Press, an imprint of The Haworth Press, Inc., 2003, pp. 115-133. Single or multiple copies of this article are available for a fee from The Haworth Document Delivery Service [1-800-HAWORTH, 9:00 a.m. - 5:00 p.m. (EST). E-mail address: getinfo@haworthpressinc.com].

115

ing monies to specific programs for specific needs. The intensity of providing and improving the delivery of services has overshadowed building connectedness across organizations and systems. Service has been the major goal and intense effort has gone into maximizing opportunities and measuring effects through service frequency. Over the past several years, new funding incentives have provided the opportunity for new collaboratives. This article describes an innovative collaboration between the Idaho Department of Health and Welfare (IDHW) and Eastern Washington University (EWU) and the unique directions and support that a university/agency partnership can provide for both organizations. Key features of this collaboration include shifts in funding and staffing strategies that contributed to more flexible services and increased levels of collaboration between IDHW, EWU and other community and state organizations and institutions. This article describes how funding can be viewed as a tool to increase the level of collaboration between systems, thus potentially leading to a breakdown of the traditional service delivery system. Finally, this article describes how an agency/higher education partnership played a key role in documenting the success of a school based program in meeting the emergency assistance needs of children and families, and how program evaluation, like funding requirements, can provide a supportive role in building collaborative relationships. *[Article copies available for a fee from The Haworth Document Delivery Service: 1-800-HAWORTH. E-mail address: <getinfo@haworthpressinc.com> Website: <http://www.HaworthPress.com> © 2003 by The Haworth Press, Inc. All rights reserved.]*

KEYWORDS. Social policy evaluation, collaboration, community development, child welfare, empowerment evaluation

Controversy and political pressure starting in the 1960s have led child welfare agencies "progressively to confine their attention to abused and neglected children" (Schorr, 2000). Currently, the political climate seems to "blame the helping professions and their service systems for their failures demanding greater accountability and threatening reductions in these professions resources and supports" (Hooper-Briar & Lawson, 1996). As a result, whether in policymaking, program development, or direct practice, those providing services to the most vulnerable families and children do so in an environment of constant change, limited resources, competing and sometimes conflicting expectations from a multitude of stakeholders (Tracy & Pine, 2000). The intensity of service delivery under these circumstances has overshadowed building connectedness among programs, and especially across service and education systems.

Historically, the formal child welfare system has not relied on informal helping networks or formalized relationships with other agencies to deliver services. Interactions with other service providers have been limited to making referrals, not collaboration. Social worker roles have been narrowly defined and generally guided by agency rather than family's needs. These agency tendencies toward inflexibility and rigid role definitions have helped create a service delivery system that appears unfriendly and non-responsive to families (Johnson, 1996).

Proponents of integrated services believe that poor education, health, and social outcomes for children result in part from the inability of the current service systems to respond in a timely, coordinated and comprehensive fashion to the multiple and interconnected needs of children and their families (David and Lucille Packard Foundation, 1992). Recently, however, we have seen the emergence of innovative, collaborative projects designed to expand the array of services and options available to populations at risk. Bailey and Koney (1996) found that ". . . public policy is beginning to reflect the importance of interorganizational community-based collaboration as a strategy for service delivery and resource maximization." This trend follows reforms in the 1970s and 80s, in which schools, child welfare and children's mental health began to fracture the categorical mold (Waldvogel, 2000, Franklin & Streeter, 1995, David and Lucille Packard Foundation, 1992). Organizations are discovering that by pooling resources their efforts are maximized, service duplication is minimized, and cross program understanding is increased, leading to improved service delivery. Additionally, shifts in funding sources and requirements have prompted states to seek collaborative partners and to experiment with creative programming to improve child welfare services outcomes.

This article will describe just such an innovative collaboration between the Idaho Department of Health and Welfare (IDHW), Eastern Washington University (EWU) and ninety Idaho school districts. The goals of this collaboration are to serve families in emergency situations in order to (1) provide increased safety and well being for children; (2) increase the learning readiness of children; and (3) increase family self-reliance. Key features of this collaboration include shifts in funding and staffing strategies that contribute to more flexible services, which better meet the needs of child welfare families. We will highlight how shifting and blending funding facilitated increasing levels of collaboration between IDHW and other agencies or institutions. This article will describe how new ways of integrating funding sources and how development of programmatic links between organizations with different roles have led to higher levels of collaboration that have affected the purpose and values of partnering systems. Finally, this article will describe the evolution of an agency/higher education partnership, which played a key role in documenting the success of this program in meeting the emergency assistance needs of children and families.

THE BEGINNING:
ESTABLISHING A IV-E FUNDED CONTRACT
TO DEVELOP PROFESSIONAL COMPETENCIES

In 1993, a relationship between IDHW and EWU was established for the purpose of providing stipend supported, MSW-level education for social work students committed to careers in child welfare. This traditional agency/university contract was funded by Title IV-E of the Social Security Act. This agreement brought together two organizations with differing goals, but similar missions–to improve service to children in the foster care system and their families. Figure 1 below shows the beginning of what would become a strong partnership.

INTEGRATION OF FUNDING STREAMS:
FROM CONTRACT TO PARTNERSHIP

In 1996, IDHW was under extreme political pressure to rapidly implement a restrictive package of state and federally mandated welfare reform policies and self-reliance supports, which had the potential of negatively impacting the child welfare system. This pressure for reform coincided with a hiring freeze and other efforts to downsize state government, including a prohibition on financing stipends for employees.

Concern regarding potential increases in numbers of child protection referrals, and a "no growth" child welfare infrastructure heightened the need for IDHW to develop partnerships with a broad range of community agencies, schools, informal sources of help, and families themselves (Waldfogel, 2000). With IDHW's emphasis on self-reliance and hiring restrictions, the IV-E stipend program no longer supported the agency's strategic direction. Thus, IDHW and EWU were required to renegotiate their relationship. Both parties were motivated to redefine their agreement to (1) continue providing relevant

FIGURE 1. IV-E Funding for IDHW/EWU Agreement

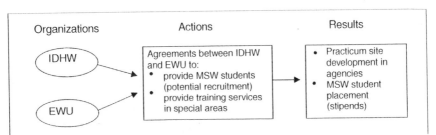

field-based learning experiences for MSW students as a recruitment and retention strategy; (2) provide training for agency staff and students on topics of significant importance to changing child welfare practice; (3) explore new methods of service delivery to vulnerable children and families, particularly through community development in rural areas; and (4) expand IDHW service capacities through the use of university student work-study resources.

In a designated frontier state like Idaho, the impacts of welfare reform could be predicted; as categorical funds dried up, community resources would be asked to fill the gap. Unfortunately, like other rural states, Idaho lacked the community resources to respond quickly and effectively to the new policies. EWU had a longstanding mission to promote rural community development practice and the resources and keen interest in studying the impact of reform on families. This formed the basis of a new partnership agreement.

One barrier to solidifying the revised partnership was the continued reliance on Title IV-E funds. Title IV-E's exclusive emphasis on foster care and adoption specialization no longer fit with the direction of Idaho's welfare reform-driven, child welfare practice. In Idaho's rural offices with staffs of one to ten persons, broad-based child welfare services could not realistically be delivered by foster care and adoption specialists, which had been the emphasis of the IV-E funding. Staff needed a generalist preparation, which emphasized prevention, early intervention, community mobilization and family preservation, in order to protect the under-resourced child welfare system from being flooded with the investigations, foster placements, terminations and adoptions that were anticipated under welfare reform.

Not only was IDHW politically restricted from continuing to finance student stipends, there was also recognition that Title IV-E funds were too restrictive to finance the strategic direction the revised partnership needed to take. EWU offered to use its student work-study mechanism as a vehicle for the partnership to begin experimenting with the delivery of community-based, emergency assistance services. IDHW agreed to pay MSW students placed in agency programs using Title IV-A funds. In turn, students were allowed to use their agency work-study sites as their field practicum sites. EWU continued to provide the work-study students a IV-E focused education and IV-E funded supervision. The blended funding arrangement provided the partnership with more flexibility regarding the range of work in which students could participate.

At about this same time, IDHW was concluding a successful pilot project with the Boise School District called the Community Resources For Families Project. In this project, child protection staff had been co-located in schools and been given the assignment to do child abuse prevention and early intervention work. These staff had access to flexible Title IV-A funds to provide at-risk families with resources necessary to prevent them from entering the child welfare or public welfare systems. IDHW and EWU were both intrigued with the model and its potential for reconfiguring the child welfare safety net in preparation for welfare reform. The partners agreed to replicate and evaluate the model, substituting MSW students paid by IV-A funds in place of child welfare staff. IDHW and EWU solicited a third partner, the Post Falls school District to participate in the replication project.

The partnership agreement and the MSW student learning contracts outlined the assessment, treatment and crises response services to be provided by the students. Supervision was provided by EWU child welfare (IV-E) field coordinators. Student placement was planned sequentially: Foundation (first year) students were placed with IDHW to gain an understanding of the complexities of child welfare practice. Advanced year (second year) interns were placed in the District's elementary schools where high percentages of students qualified for free and reduced lunch.

Ultimately, the MSW work study students proved successful in replicating the prevention/early intervention services and in the administering of the flexible IV-A Emergency Assistance funds. Additionally, partnering in the establishment of early intervention services to reduce the gap between the basic needs faced by families (housing, medical, clothing, food), and in the ability of the system to meet the needs in a timely way, showed great potential in averting families from potential referral to the child protection system. Finally, the expansion of the partnership, to include the school district as the location of child welfare service delivery, had a significant community capacity-building effect. This shift in the partnership began the movement away from a singular focus on preservice education to one of collaboration and community development. Figure 2 illustrates this change.

MOVEMENT TO NEW LEVELS OF COLLABORATION: ONE RESULT OF WELFARE REFORM

In 1997, IDHW implemented welfare reform. With welfare reform, the federal government abolished Title IV-A and replaced it with Temporary Assistance for Needy Families (TANF) funds. States that had IV-A plans and services in place prior to welfare reform were encouraged to use their welfare reform savings to maintain or expand the child welfare and family self-reliance services they already had in place. IDHW used this opportunity to enter partnerships with ninety school districts in Idaho. TANF funding was used to contract with these districts in hiring Community Resources Workers (CRW) to develop and deliver Community Resources for Families (CRFF) services

FIGURE 2. Stage 2: Using Blended Funds to Improve Service (IV-E, IV-B, TANF, Administration for Children, Youth and Families Grant)

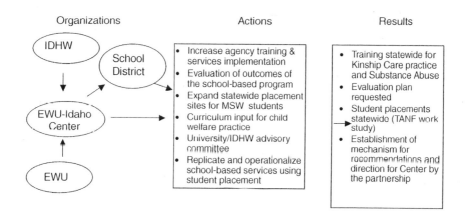

statewide. In addition, IDHW blended TANF funds with Title IV-E funds to sustain and again redirect the partnership with EWU. Using TANF funds, the Department asked EWU to work collaboratively with the districts in developing the research and evaluation component of the statewide Community Resources for Families program implementation.

Also in 1997, IDHW and EWU entered general discussions regarding the research and program development needs of IDHW, specifically related to preparation for the anticipated implementation of the Adoption and Safe Families Act, in 1998. It was during these discussions that both parties acknowledged that the partnership had grown so large that a new administrative structure was necessary to support all of the activity. As a result, the School of Social Work and IDHW created the Idaho Child Welfare Research and Training Center (EWU-Idaho Center). This Center, funded by IDHW and staffed through the partnership by EWU School of Social Work, blended several funding sources to maintain the previously described work and to add services that would support ASFA implementation. In particular, Title IV-E, IV-B, and TANF were used to support the Center. Additionally, the Center was successful in writing an ACYF (Administration for Children, Youth, and Families) grant to support a statewide Kinship Care Training Initiative for Idaho. Thus, the relationship between IDHW and EWU School of Social Work continued to change: the diversification of funding brought new goals into the partnership, and the establishment of the EWU-Idaho Center brought new voices to the decision making process in IDHW.

One of the ways that IDHW envisioned reaching their important goals of getting appropriate services to the most needy children and families was to expand the successful school-based pilot programs into a statewide initiative. These programs offered several advantages for the Department. First, the partnership included a mechanism for early identification of the most distressed families through the needs manifested by children in the school environment. Second, the pilot programs enhanced the relationships IDHW had with schools and local communities. And third, by passing TANF funding through to schools to subsequently hire social workers, IDHW had a new post-welfare reform infrastructure.

It is important here to describe briefly the Community Resources for Families program as it has come to be developed in more than ninety school districts across the State of Idaho. With program coordination and funding provided by IDHW, local school districts hire Community Resource Workers (CRW'S) to serve local elementary schools. These CRW's receive referrals from principals, counselors and teachers for children who are exhibiting signs of distress leading to school failure and/or social problems. Referral reasons include unmet basic needs such as lack of food, clothing, or shelter, as well as poor school performance for unknown reasons, poor school attendance, and behavioral issues that defy school interventions. In many cases, family stressors are the foundation of the signs of need, and these stressors often lead to problems in the child's' attendance, behavior, and academics. The CRW'S are social workers who work closely with families to resolve issues that threaten the safety or learning readiness of children, including helping families connect with community resources. During the 1999-2000 school year, 5,918 families were referred to and served by the CRFF program.

We describe this program briefly here because it served as a springboard for further collaboration between IDHW and Eastern Washington University. Figure 3 below illustrates how this program promotes collaboration between the partners; not only are various funding streams blended to provide monies for the schools, but the service model itself provides collaborative links between the community and agencies at state, district, and local levels to support families, and between the agency, teachers, and families to support children.

STAGE 4:
MOVING BEYOND FUNDING:
ALIGNING VALUES TO ADVANCE COLLABORATION

The expansion to a statewide model of the Community Resources for Families program precipitated IDHW to expand the role of its partnership with the EWU-Idaho Center as a means of addressing more specifically program evalu-

FIGURE 3. Community Resources for Families Program

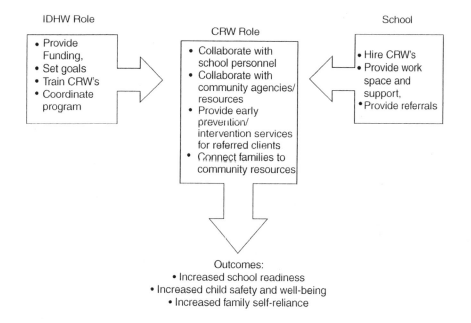

IDHW Role

- Provide Funding,
- Set goals
- Train CRW's
- Coordinate program

CRW Role

- Collaborate with school personnel
- Collaborate with community agencies/ resources
- Provide early prevention/ intervention services for referred clients
- Connect families to community resources

School

- Hire CRW's
- Provide work space and support,
- Provide referrals

Outcomes:
- Increased school readiness
- Increased child safety and well-being
- Increased family self-reliance

ation. After successfully negotiating the means to blend funds to support the program and the partnership with EWU, IDHW recognized the need to work within the outcome measurement expectations set by the Adoptions and Safe Families Act (ASFA). The ASFA outcome measurements go beyond counting the service frequencies of agency personnel; in addition to such measures, ASFA also looks at quality of life issues, including success at school, as a measure of program success.

The ASFA outcome expectations, though not a source of funding, motivated the Department to seek new ways of complying with the mandate, in order to sustain current funding levels. And here, IDHW had an enigma; it was in the midst of creating a computer tracking system for the state-wide school based program that collected data on service frequencies based on previously recognized reporting and documentation needs, rather than on the client outcomes expected by ASFA. Thus, IDHW turned to an established partner, the EWU-Idaho Center, to collaborate around developing outcome measures.

This move to a new, problem-solving level of collaboration between the organizations brought an interesting sidelight. Partners can bring to collaboration differing orientations and values around a common goal or mission. The

School of Social Work at EWU is characterized by an empowerment orientation and promotes a strength-based approach to working with families. This is taught in their curriculum and is valued as an integrating knowledge and skill in their students. IDHW had earlier adopted a family-centered practice approach. However, it was using a traditional service provider tracking evaluation to measure its impact. Thus IDHW was blunting or negating a consistent family-centered approach. The inclusion of an empowerment evaluation model* into the school program resulted in several role shifts and attendant tensions. (*Empowerment evaluation is the use of evaluation concepts, techniques, and findings to foster improvement and self-determination. It employs both qualitative and quantitative methodologies (Empowerment Evaluation, 2000).)

The first role change occurred when program managers and supervisors were asked by the evaluator to define what the program was supposed to accomplish. This challenged them to move from a service provision and implementation role to a program design role. The focus shifted from seeking to meet client needs in an efficient manner to helping clients reach individually valued outcomes. This shift was felt at every level of the program, for at the field level it asked CRW'S to set goals *with* clients rather than *for* them, and to measure success in individually valued outcomes. And, it asked for clear goals against which to measure progress.

A second role change occurred around data collection itself. The relationship between IDHW supervisors and field workers had been built on a service model; what was valued was a linear connection between what the database asked for, in the form of the case file, and what the field worker actually did. The empowerment evaluation model asked field staff to build relationships between themselves and their client such that the worker could document actual changes in client behaviors as a result of service. This began to challenge the role of the supervisor from one of compliance monitoring to one of problem solving around revising services that are not effectively impacting behavior changes and client-centered outcomes.

At another level, the empowerment evaluation process asked program line staff to refine their roles in maintaining standards of best practice. This applied specifically to development of a statewide informed consent process when working with clients. The evaluation component and its required attention to human subject considerations challenged the organization to develop and apply a consistent policy. Again supervisors were faced with role redefinition/clarification as they became part of the evaluative process in assuring informed consent.

These role challenges generated discussions between the new demands of the evaluation component and the conceptions of practice that were currently in place. In this manner, evaluation itself functioned as a precipitator of change, supported by the potential of new funding requirements *for practice* in the near future. In effect, adding the evaluation component helped the collaboration function at a new level, a level at which organizational and philosophical values started to frame how the collaboration might proceed. Figure 4 below illustrates several of the differing values brought to light by the move toward this new level of collaboration.

The tensions between aligning the funding parameters (i.e.: TANF, IV-E ASFA) as represented by evaluation and the current practices around the school program implementation and monitoring by IDHW led to adoption of a new strategy for how the collaboration could serve the program. Each of the seven regions of the state is distinct not only in IDHW leadership, but also in the political and environmental context. Thus, the EWU-Idaho Center evaluators worked with each region to choose a pilot site that would represent region-specific outcomes. In this way the pilot sites facilitated deeper relationships and understandings between the Center staff and supervisors and managers at the district level. In addition, service data collected through an empowerment orientation started showing significant gains on the part of clients, gains that were previously intuitively sensed but not documented.

For example, one of the pilot sites found a close correlation between the ratings on tools used by parents or guardians to judge a child's progress, and the

FIGURE 4. Operative Values of IDHW Program Staff and Empowerment Evaluation Model

Value Criteria	Operational Values	
	IDHW	Empowerment Evaluation
Valued Data	Frequency counts showing aggregated decreases in need for IDHW or CPS services	Individual client data around goals and needs with resultant services
Valued Goals	assure safety of children through assessment and referral process	Empower all constituencies through self-evaluative processes
Valued Processes	Delivery of services via traditional contact and referral system	Development of supports and delivery of services through collaborating with teachers, parents, children around goal setting
Valued Questions	Determining how much or often services are effective	Determining how to best serve individual clients

classroom teacher's rating of that same child. Further, the process of collecting the data seemed to support the progress; there were significant pre-post findings for the children identified in the pilot. This data illustrated for the IDHW program supervisors as a collective group that school data could be used to support claims of program effectiveness. It also validated the perceptions of parents or guardians as part of a measurement process for documenting improvement in their children. Another pilot illustrated how the program seems to impact school data directly. This pilot showed significant changes pre-post in how parents rated their needs on nine areas of family well being and safety. In addition, the children from the families who showed significant changes also showed important increases in school performance. Again, this pilot data became a catalyst for helping IDHW program supervisors envision different possibilities for data collection around the program, and prompted more of a collaborative orientation toward working with schools around measurement criteria.

The results of the pilot data precipitated progress in advancing the school/agency/university collaboration in the following way: (1) school data became seen as desirable and obtainable; (2) the pilot outcome data suggested that changes in practice could in fact lead to positive and documented program results, and (3) the discussion around the usefulness of evaluation changed from one of defensiveness to one of cautious curiosity. Most importantly, the pilot studies seemed to lay the path for an important opportunity to further the collaborative partnership.

STATE FUNDING PRIORITIES: ALWAYS A FACTOR

After the first year of collecting data for the Community Resources for Families program, funding for the program was jeopardized by shifting priorities within the State budget. In an effort to substantiate the usefulness of the program for continued funding, IDHW regional managers and supervisors turned to its collaborative partner, the EWU-Idaho Center, to document program effectiveness. The request by the IDHW to collect outcome and effectiveness data allowed the Center to give voice to some of its goals and values in the evaluation design. It also for the first time allowed the schools to become more of a partner in the effort, as school data became an important part of the effectiveness ratings. In effect, the prospect of losing funding from the legislative process promoted a wider vision of the program and the collaboration. And, the fact that the resulting evaluation effort validated the strong progress made by students and families in the program served to solidify a collaboration that had been mostly instrumental in the past.

Figure 5 below illustrates the collaborative goals that are now potentially involved in the statewide, school-based Community Resources for Families program. Although the connection between IDHW and the schools remains a one-way action at this point, discussions have begun about how to partner with the schools in setting goals around the program.

THE INFLUENCE OF FUNDING
ON COLLABORATIVE PARTNERSHIPS:
BUILDING AN UNDERSTANDING

The collaboration between IDHW and EWU-Idaho Center has gone through several stages, beginning with the utilization of Title IV-E funds to support child welfare employees interested in an advanced degree in social work and to recruit MSW students into the field of child welfare. The application of various funding streams has led to changes in the relationships between the partners and to future possibilities unforeseen during the beginning stages. A framework developed by Franklin and Streeter (1995) has been adapted to describe the evolution of the collaboration between IDHW and EWU-Idaho Center. This framework also provides a means to look at next steps in terms of further collaboration development.

Figures 6 and 7 below show how the relationship has moved from a level of interaction most appropriately called "informal relations" to a level of interaction that is thoroughly "partnership" and verging on "collaboration." The various categories of the chart illustrate some of the possible criteria by

FIGURE 5. Stage 3: Using Block Grants to Achieve Common Goals

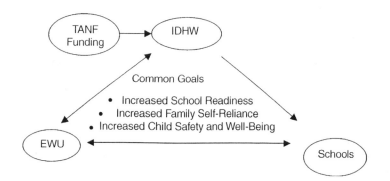

which a developing relationship may be assessed. An important point for the current discussion is the funding criteria; it can be seen that as the funding has diversified, the relationship has become more complex. This may be a critical area for program development involving multiple partners, for funding streams themselves can be seen to include mandates that force partners into new roles.

The dark boxes in Figure 6 indicate the type of relationship that existed between IDHW and the EWU School of Social Work at the contractual phase. The formal agreements that were created allowed accountability in transferring funds between organizations. In all other respects, the relationship can be characterized as an informal arrangement to provide services to children and families.

Figure 7 below illustrates the somewhat dramatic changes that occurred during the period from 1994-2000. First, the diversity of funding steams used to support the Community Resources for Families program, which became the spearhead for the collaboration, required formal agreements at several levels, particularly between independent school boards and IDHW. In this area, the relationships came to function as a true collaboration.

Second, the planning aspect of the relationship has moved significantly in the direction of collaboration. IDHW maintains a focused agenda in terms of the use of funds, although that agenda has broadened to include increasing the school readiness of children, which is part of the agenda from the educational partners. A third area of movement has been around training. Training needs have been negotiated between IDHW and EWU-Idaho Center, with each partner taking a beginning responsibility for appropriate training roles.

The most dramatic change has been in the innovative use of funding to advance service provision to children and families. As described above, there have been distinct stages in this area, with increased diversity of funding generally leading to increased complexity of relationships. A final and more subtle change has been in the sharing of values between the agencies involved. In particular, partners have come together around the kinds of measurements that will show program effectiveness and have learned to celebrate progress across several scales.

The above figure illustrates key points in the development: from informal commitment in an agency/university agreement; to the use of students in a replication project implementing school-based services; to the introduction of

FIGURE 6. Continuum of Linkages Between Agencies (IDHW, School of Social Work, Public Schools): Bolded Cells Indicate Current Development (After Franklin & Streeter, 1995)

The Beginning Stage: Relationships Under Title IV-E Funding Services for Interns(1995)

| Implementation Factors → | 5 Levels of Relationships between Agencies | | | | |
	Informal Relations	Coordination	Partnership	Collaboration	Integration
Commitment to Formal Agreements	Little commitment required	Some commitment to formal agreements	commitment to formal agreements required	Formal agreements between boards and state	Formal agreements between boards, state, and local agencies
Planning	Planning done by individual agencies	Some common planning done by agencies	Formal agreements based on one agency's agenda	Formal agreements based on client needs	Comprehensive planning at state level with local level input
Training	Training done by individual agencies	Training needs set by agencies together	Training of agencies' staff on roles/function of partners	Ongoing and intensive interprofessional education	Ongoing interprofessional education and inter-disciplinary teamwork
Funding	Single source of funding outside of agencies (IV-E)	multiple sources of funding outside of agencies (IV-E; IV-B)	Additional funding within agencies for new services(IV-E; IV-B; TANF)	Additional funding from agencies and community	Additional required funding leads to re-structuring agencies
Value Sharing	Recognized but not shared values	Values shared to pursue individual agendas	Values blended to pursue individual agendas	Values shared to increase services	Value sharing leads to restructuring of agendas

FIGURE 7. The Current Stage: Relationships Utilizing Blended Funding and Block Grants (Fall, 2000)

Implementation Factor	5 Levels of Relationships Between Agencies				
	Informal Relations	Coordination	Partnership	Collaboration	Integration
Commitment	Little commitment required	Some commitment to formal agreements	Commitment to formal agreements required	Formal agreements between boards and state	Formal agreements between boards, state, and local agencies
Planning	Planning done by individual agencies	Some common planning done by agencies	Formal agreements based on one agency's agenda	Formal agreements based on client needs	Comprehensive planning at state level with local level input
Training	Training done by individual agencies	Training needs set by agencies together	Training of agencies' staff on roles/function of partners	Ongoing and intensive interprofessional education	Ongoing interprofessional education and inter-disciplinary teamwork
Funding	Single source of funding outside of agencies (IV-E)	Multiple sources of funding outside of agencies (IV-E; IV-B)	Additional funding within agencies for new services (IV-E; IV-B; TANF)	Additional funding from agencies and community	Additional required funding leads to restructuring agencies
Value Sharing	Recognized but not shared values	Values shared to pursue individual agendas	Values blended to pursue individual agendas	Values shared to increase services	Value sharing leads to restructuring of agendas

new funding streams (TANF); and finally the influence of pilot site replication on the implementation of the statewide, Community Resources for Families Program. We can summarize this development as follows:

1. The commitment between partners proceeded the actual practice. Formal, mainly financial, agreements were a major reason for moving to a collaborative model, and those agreements are soundly in place.
2. Collaborative planning is still a desired goal of this partnership. At present, the single funding source–TANF funds–dictates this particular program agenda. However, current indications are that collaborative planning will occur, especially around the evaluation portion of the agreements.
3. Training needs are currently set (in collaboration) by two of three partners, the EWU-Idaho Center and IDHW. Public school personnel are not yet partners in training, although they sporadically attend trainings planned by the Center. Identification of cross-agency training agendas remains to be accomplished.
4. Funding sources have been blended brilliantly to produce the current level of program collaboration. It is recognized that additional development will depend upon availability of collaborative funding sources.
5. Value sharing has proceeded quickly within the last year, due in part to the influence of funding requirements for outcome evaluations (ASFA) and the entry of an outside evaluator into the program. IDHW foresees a future that includes value sharing among partners, and movement is underway to accomplish that goal.
6. Empowerment evaluation, which helps individuals and clients at all levels of service to become clear about goals important to them, can function as a tool to increase collaboration between institutions. Traditional evaluation methods, which seek only to identify program effects, does not seem to serve this purpose.

CONCLUSION

This article has tracked the key role that funding has had on an agency/university partnership in the development of an innovative program designed to meet the needs of children and families following significant devolution funding shifts. We have looked at how a program can move from mainly a status of informal relations, in spite of formal financial agreements, to a much more developed partnership verging on collaboration. Federal policy and funding shifts are seen as a major contributor to the development of advanced relationships between the Idaho Department of Health and Welfare and the Eastern

Washington University School of Social Work. Other major contributors to the development of a successful and innovative program have been the creativity and professional pursuits of IDHW staff and EWU School of Social Work faculty who serve as staff for the EWU-Idaho Center. The movement toward high levels of collaboration was accelerated by the addition of an evaluation component working through conflicting value orientations. This has led to clearer program goals and the opportunity to look at practice through a different values orientation.

This article is in effect a celebration of the efforts of IDHW personnel to work through the maze of funding shifts for the benefit of children in the State of Idaho. The impact funding shifts can have on practices is also positive; human services provision remains quintessentially human, and the dedication of professionals from three organizations, the EWU-Idaho Center, the Idaho Department of Health and Welfare and the public schools have combined to turn funding challenges into services opportunities.

REFERENCES

Bailey, D., & Koney, D.M. (1996) Interorganizational community-based collaboratives: A strategic response to shape the social work agenda. *Social Work*, 41, #6, 602-611.

Casey Outcomes and Decision-Making Project. (1998). *Assessing outcomes in child welfare services: Principles, concepts, and a framework of core indicators.* American Humane Association: Englewood, CO: Author.

Franklin, C., & Streeter, C. L. (1995). School reform: Linking public schools with human services. *Social Work*, 40, #6, 773-781.

Guba, E. G., & Lincoln, Y. S. (1989). *Fourth generation evaluation.* Newbury Park: Sage.

Health Canada. *Guide to project evaluation: A participatory approach.* National Clearinghouse on Family Violence: Ottawa, Ontario: Author.

Hooper-Briar, K., & Lawson, H., Eds.(1996) *Expanding partnerships for vulnerable children, youth, and families.* Council on Social Work Education, Alexandria, Virginia.

Hopkins, K, Mudrick, N., & Rudolph, C. (1999). Impact of university/agency partnerships in child welfare on organizations, workers, and work activities. *Child Welfare*, 78, #6, 749-773.

House, E.R., & Howe, K. R. (2000). Deliberative democratic evaluation. *New Directions for Evaluation* 85, 3-12.

Johnson, I., (1996) Child welfare agencies, families, and communities: A vital partnership. *Expanding Partnerships for Vulnerable Children, Youth, and Families.* Council on Social Work Education, Alexandria, Virginia.

Madison, A.M. (2000). Language in defining social problems and in evaluating social programs. *New Directions for Evaluation.* 86, 17-28.

Petr, C.G. (1998). *Social work with children and their families.* Oxford University Press.

Rosenfeld, L.B., Richman, J.M., & Bowen, G.L., (2000). *Child and Adolescent Social Work Journal*, 17, #3, 205-227.

Schalock, R.L. (1995). *Outcome-based evaluation.* New York: Plenum Press.

Schorr, A., (2000). The bleak prospect for public child welfare. *The Social Service Review*, 74, #1, 124-136.

Smrekar, C., (1998). The organizational and political threats to school-linked integrated services, *Educational Policy*, 12, #3, 284-304.

Tracy, E., & Pine, B., (2000). Child welfare education and training: Future trends and influences. *Child Welfare*, 79, #1, 93-113.

The David & Lucille Packard Foundation (1992) School-linked services, *The Future of Children*, 2, #1, Center for the Future of Children.

Waldfogel, J., (2000) Reforming child protective services. *Child Welfare*, 79, #1, 43-57.

The California Collaboration:
A Competency-Based
Child Welfare Curriculum Project
for Master's Social Workers

Sherrill Clark

SUMMARY. This article documents the Title IV-E child welfare social work project of the California Social Work Education Center (CalSWEC): The establishment and ongoing support of collaborative arrangements among 58 California counties, the California State Department of Social Services, and all of the California graduate social work schools. The primary goal of this collaboration is to produce MSWs who will commit to helping disadvantaged children and families in publicly supported child welfare services. The project model contains five interdependent components: a competency-based curriculum, financial support for students, development of instructional materials, active participation among public child welfare agencies and the universities, and evaluation.

This paper focuses on the collaborative curriculum development process. Evolving arrangements among stakeholders are described here in terms of the reciprocal adjustment of curriculum development and field

Sherrill Clark, PhD, MSW, is Research Specialist and formerly the Executive Director, California Social Work Education Center, University of California, Berkeley, School of Social Welfare, 120 Haviland Hall, Berkeley, CA 94720-7400 (E-mail: sjclark@uclink.berkeley.edu).

[Haworth co-indexing entry note]: "The California Collaboration: A Competency-Based Child Welfare Curriculum Project for Master's Social Workers." Clark, Sherrill. Co-published simultaneously in *Journal of Behavior in the Social Environment* (The Haworth Social Work Practice Press, an imprint of The Haworth Press, Inc.) Vol. 7, No. 1/2, 2003, pp. 135-157; and: *Charting the Impacts of University-Child Welfare Collaboration* (ed: Katharine Briar-Lawson, and Joan Levy Zlotnik) The Haworth Social Work Practice Press, an imprint of The Haworth Press, Inc., 2003, pp. 135-157. Single or multiple copies of this article are available for a fee from The Haworth Document Delivery Service [1-800-HAWORTH, 9:00 a.m. - 5:00 p.m. (EST). E-mail address: getinfo@haworthpressinc.com].

and classroom instruction to prepare MSWs for public child welfare careers. *[Article copies available for a fee from The Haworth Document Delivery Service: 1-800-HAWORTH. E-mail address: <getinfo@haworthpressinc.com> Website: <http://www.HaworthPress.com> © 2003 by The Haworth Press, Inc. All rights reserved.]*

KEYWORDS. University-agency partnerships, curriculum development, Title IV-E funding, public child welfare education

INTRODUCTION

The following article describes a 10 year collaborative public agency-university child welfare social work project in process, one of the first of its kind to utilize Title IV-E funding for MSW education[1]. The California Deans and Directors of Graduate Schools of Social Work and the California Welfare Directors Association created CalSWEC to encourage Master's level social work graduates in the state to prepare for careers in the publicly supported social services [Grossman et al. 1992]. Since 1992, the ongoing collaborative arrangements have produced more than 1100 MSWs who are committed to helping disadvantaged children and families in publicly supported child welfare services.

The goal of this collaboration's use of Title IV-E funding is to produce MSWs who will commit to helping disadvantaged children and their families in foster care or at risk of placement. It is thought that infusing social work values and methods will ultimately refocus the child welfare system on the development and maintenance of healthy families and safe children. The Center's initial objectives involved the creation of a program of financial aid for students linked to a competency-based curriculum developed jointly by educators and professionals in the public agencies and with employment requirements to be met upon graduation.

The project model contains five interdependent components: financial support for students, a competency-based curriculum, program and curriculum evaluation, resource support for the development of instructional materials, and active participation among public child welfare agencies and the universities. This paper focuses on the keystone quality assurance piece: the curriculum.

The first part of this article describes the need over a decade for child welfare workers in California. Next, the article describes the joint agency-university curriculum development process from 1991 to 1996 and the ongoing modification process in terms of a tool for strengthening the collaboration. Collaborative arrangements among stakeholders are described here in terms of evolving reciprocal adjustments of classroom and field curriculum and field instruction. The definition of a competency-based curriculum, the process of selecting a diverse advisory group of child welfare experts, a description of the methodology, and the results of the curriculum development process are included here. Initial similarities and differences between practitioners' and faculties' views about what is essential for inclusion in a graduate child welfare social work program are noted. Then, how those views evolved as stakeholders gained more experience with the curriculum is discussed, emphasizing how this joint development process strengthens understanding and shared responsibility.

By using competencies, rather than mandating specific courses in child welfare, a step-wise approach was successfully used to strengthen the public child welfare social work curriculum. Next steps are suggested for modification of the curriculum as another opportunity.[2] Finally, the limitations of this model for social work education development and recommendations for improvement are discussed.

ESTABLISHING THE NEED FOR MSWs IN CHILD WELFARE

Deaths or injuries of children often focus intense scrutiny on public child welfare programs. These incidents reflect the pressure of caseloads that are rapidly increasing in numbers and acuity, while resources are diminished. Not infrequently, however, workers who have committed serious practice errors have been poorly educated for the complex skills associated with child welfare practice. In several cases in other states, departments of social services have been found deficient in observing legal and professional practice standards. States have been sued and resulting consent decrees have included requirements for upgrading child welfare staff, showing hiring preferences for persons with human services bachelors' degrees or Masters in Social Work [NASW 1989b]. However, the kinds of consent decrees that have the widest range, i.e., those which seek to reform large child welfare systems themselves, often have negative effects on resources. That is to say, states focus resources on compliance under consent decrees rather than on upgrading the professional skills of the workforce [Blome, 1998].

Historically, social work has been the leading deliverer of services in child welfare practice, but professionally trained graduate social workers have not predominated. A national study done in the 1970s indicated in a sample of 38 states and the District of Columbia that only 9 percent of child welfare workers had an MSW [Shyne & Schroeder, 1978]. A decade later, a study of 16 states showed the percentage had risen to 13 percent [Lieberman et al., 1988].

The need for MSWs is particularly profound with respect to professionals who are members of ethnic and racial groups, particularly in a state that contains one-third of the immigrants in the United States [Wong, 2001]. These changes in California's population require more staff from the underrepresented ethnic groups and more bilingual workers. Child welfare staffs do not represent the same ethnic mix as the poor, recent immigrant, and refugee populations [Tatara, 1991; Harris et al., 1993]. Bilingual and bicultural social workers are in short supply and many of them must finish baccalaureate degrees before they can take advantage of the Title IV-E MSW program.

Child welfare jobs are very difficult and emotionally taxing. The relationship between educational opportunities for workers and the ability to handle the distress of these difficult jobs is just now beginning to be examined [Dickinson & Perry, 1998]. Contrary to popular opinion, child welfare jobs are among the most complicated and call for a wide range of knowledge and skill. It is for this reason that professional social work is particularly suited for this type of practice.

At least one study has demonstrated some relevance of professional social work education to child welfare practice [Booz-Allen 1987]. Another study has found that MSWs were most successful in the delivery of substitute services, including "more successful in finding adoptive homes for the children assigned to them than were other groups of workers" [Olsen & Holmes, 1982: 99]. A more recent analysis has found that for children placed in foster care, caseworkers with a social work degree (BSW or MSW) were significantly more likely to carry out "a permanent plan within three years than those without a social work degree" [Albers, Reilly et al., 1993: 337].

THE DEVELOPMENT OF COMPETENCIES FOR MSW CHILD WELFARE PRACTICE: BACKGROUND

Prior to the collaboration in 1990, each institution stayed in its own camp. Agency staff were skeptical of the capabilities of new MSW graduates to perform the necessary tasks for public social work practice. By the same token, faculty were not convinced that social workers in public agencies would be able to practice according to professional standards.

Consequently, it was important for the schools of social work to show good faith. The deans did this by passing in each school, a common mission statement emphasizing preparation for practice in publicly-supported social services serving poor and disadvantaged clients. The county welfare directors as a group demonstrated their effort by participating in and approving the competencies for practice in public child welfare and are active members of the board and its committees.

The design and structure of graduate curricula are the province of each faculty and a variety of curriculum models may be effective. By delineating a basic set of educational knowledge and skill competencies and basic values that the schools could adopt as curriculum objectives in child welfare, CalSWEC hoped to assure an appropriate level of consistency in MSW training for child welfare throughout the state of California with the minimum amount of interference.

From 1991 to 1996, CalSWEC worked with the schools of social work to integrate the child welfare knowledge and value competencies with existing MSW practice, policy, research methods, and human development courses wherever possible. For the more specific skill-based competencies, CalSWEC offered instructional support to assist schools in developing field placements and delivering integrative field seminars mostly in the second year to cover the more specific core child welfare skills and methods. Assistance to the schools and the county social services departments in the collaborative implementation of curriculum for the education and training of MSW child welfare workers remains a key function of CalSWEC.[3]

Key to the care and tending of an active collaboration is having persons who are well versed in more than one institutional language and able to translate one for the other. For the CalSWEC project, each school is allotted one project coordinator whose job it is to act as a boundary spanner between the practice field and the university. These project coordinators, some of whom have been with the project for eight years, are a unique form of academic and practice expert.

THE REASONS FOR USING COMPETENCIES TO INFLUENCE CURRICULUM DEVELOPMENT

Competent means being "properly or well qualified; capable; adequate for the purposes defined" [Berube, 1985]. Competency further implies expertise, proficiency, and mastery of a particular skill or body of knowledge. The idea of competency-based social work education is not new [Gambrill, 1983; Freisen, 1986; Hughes & Rycus, 1989; Institute for Human Services, 1987; Tabbert & Sullivan, 1988; Wolfe, 1989; Pecora et al., 1990; LeCroy, 1990; Cheung et al., 1991; Maine Child Welfare Training Institute, 1991]. Without specification, the ability to know or do child welfare social work is an ambiguous, overwhelming goal for education.

A competency-based curriculum, (1) provides clear descriptions of what skills or knowledge are measured and how (including the selection of distinct outcomes chosen before the interventions begin), (2) follows progress during the intervention process, (3) employs empirical literature, and (4) applies critical thinking skills [Gambrill 1983]. A competency-based curriculum must select elements that have clear, measurable descriptions and distinct outcomes are chosen before the interventions begin. The elements must allow for the ability to follow progress during the intervention process. Empirical literature and the application of critical thinking skills are used in the development of the elements [Gambrill, 1983]. Therefore, one of the first tasks of the curriculum committee was to carefully specify the skills, knowledge and values desired by an advanced practitioner in child welfare, while using the context of the professional social work foundation.

The professional foundation, as formulated by the major accrediting body for social work education, the Council on Social Work Education, bases social work curricula on five professional foundation content areas [CSWE, 1994]. The foundation includes Human Behavior and the Social Environment, Social Welfare Policy and Services, Social Work Practice, Research, and the Field Practicum. CSWE further states: "Both levels [the baccalaureate and the master's] of social work must provide the professional foundation curriculum that contains the common body of knowledge, values, and skills of the profession. . . . The master's level of social work education must include the professional foundation content and concentration content for advanced practice in an identifiable area. [CSWE, 1994: 136]. This statement does not suggest that the development of discrete courses is the only way to address specialty programs. In fact as noted above, when CalSWEC created the competencies, the goal was to infuse the curriculum with the knowledge, skills and values needed to work with disadvantaged families and children.

The California public child welfare service delivery model includes discrete service categories based on policy specifications for the delivery of child welfare services (see, for example, the Adoptions and Safe Families Act). For several years, the distinct program areas have been: Adoptions, Emergency Response, Family Reunification, Family Maintenance, and Permanency Planning. Rather than organize social work courses around these service categories, CalSWEC developed a set of competencies that would prepare social workers for specialized practice in child welfare, yet be woven into the professional foundation content areas as described by CSWE. This competency-based curriculum does not require that specific child welfare courses be developed, but it does require problem solving among the schools and agencies to determine how to provide students experiences to enable learning in specific child welfare areas.

In fact, there has been concern for some time among professionals that what social workers are learning does not "fit the problems the problems of families most frequently encountered in child welfare" [Wiltse, 1981]. A national survey done by Lauderdale (1980) indicated that classroom instructors felt most confident about their students' knowledge regarding child welfare policy, supportive services, and legislation. The development of treatment skills in the special problems of children, while the most desired graduate course was the least frequently taught. Classroom instructors relied on the field placement experience to teach these skills to their students. The reader is left with the impression that the classroom and the field operated on two different curricula.

As it happens, very few classroom courses correspond directly to the program areas, e.g., have titles such as, *Child Abuse and Neglect* or *Child Protective Services* [Kravitz, 1991], nor should they, necessarily. To the extent that there is child welfare content in the curriculum, it is found in case examples in foundation courses or in specialized electives about the child and family. However, even specialized electives do not represent a systematic treatment of the subject of child welfare because mental health content has predominated in specialized electives about the child and family [LeCroy, 1990]. When the presence of child welfare content is not assured or treated in a comprehensive way, all students do not have equal opportunity to learn using child welfare examples. Finally, there has been little documentation of the transfer of learning process: applying classroom knowledge and skills in the field or using the field experience to enhance classroom learning.

The National Association of Public Child Welfare Administrators' survey of the collaborative efforts of public child welfare agencies and schools of social work encourages the development of competency-based assessment of practice [NAPCWA 1991]. For this curriculum effort, collaboration and specificity of curriculum elements were regarded as primary goals. CalSWEC felt that starting with the elements themselves, rather than challenging existing structures in either the university or the agency domain, a curriculum could be developed that met the needs of both professional graduate social work education and professional child welfare services. The expectation was (and is) that capable graduate social work specialists in child welfare should be skilled and knowledgeable in these competencies.

Curricula must be sensitive to changes in public policy, the distribution of client populations, available resources, and existing knowledge about what works to alleviate social problems. At the same time curricula must adhere to and promote professional values and ethics. Hence the education for professional social work practice by necessity involves collaboration between field practitioners and social work faculty. The methods chosen for the development of the child welfare curriculum allow for the fact that people already have ways of doing things that work for them, but that new ways of educating child welfare workers must also be developed. The first steps were to select a panel of experts conversant in various aspects of child welfare as well as with the process of social work field education and to mail them a questionnaire containing a list of competencies.

THE MAILED SURVEY: METHODOLOGY AND RESULTS

The main source for our original competency list was a document entitled, *Individual Training Needs Assessment for Child Welfare Caseworkers*, developed by Ronald C. Hughes and Judith Rycus of the Institute for Human Services [IHS], Columbus, Ohio [IHS, 1987]. There were two additional primary sources.[4] In 1991, using the Delphi method, a mailed survey consisting of 126 suggested competencies was sent to the panel of 30 experts [Delbeq, 1975; Lauffer, 1984]. This panel consisted of child welfare practitioners and faculty who were nominated by members of the Curriculum Committee which consisted of 3 welfare directors/practitioners and 3 deans/directors. From the mailed survey, respondents indicated which competencies were *necessary, desirable*, or *unnecessary* for public child welfare practice. The competencies on which the practitioners and the faculty agreed could be taught in the MSW curriculum and which were necessary for child welfare practice are listed in Table 1.

An interesting dichotomy developed from the mailed survey results. Faculty felt they could teach the competency areas in Table 2, but practitioners thought this was too much to expect of the schools and opted for saving these competencies for on-the-job training. Consequently these competencies, although everyone agreed they were important, were identified as "advanced" competencies that beginning social workers would have to learn on the job.

In 1991, after much review of the list of competencies by the Curriculum Committee, CalSWEC held a statewide conference to encourage regional school-agency collaborations. Over 100 child welfare practitioners and teachers attended, among them the 30 members of the panel and the members of the curriculum committee.

TABLE 1. Competencies Indicating Faculty/Practitioner Agreement

- Ethnic sensitive practice
- Understanding of basic child welfare practice
- Basic social work skills and methods
- Human development and the effect of child abuse and neglect
- Understanding interdisciplinary teamwork
- Understanding the role of the child welfare manager as team developer.

TABLE 2. Competencies Indicating Faculty/Practitioner Differences

- The legal basis for child welfare practice
- Child welfare assessment and specialized child welfare practice
- Advanced skills relating to interdisciplinary work
- Skills working with the client's community on behalf of the client and the client/family group.

One of the original conference activities consisted of a general discussion of the competencies that were important learning priorities but that were not adequately represented in the field or classroom. Following that, participants met in groups by California state region to identify regional gaps in the curriculum. Agencies and schools that shared students and field placements were asked to then make specific, local plans for curriculum development addressing these gaps. Table 3 shows the priority areas identified by these regional groups as lacking in child welfare education by California state region.

These competencies noted as gaps in the curricula of the schools of social work were discussed by the Curriculum Committee who, after a request for proposal process, then allotted funding resources for developing new curricula in those areas which could be disseminated among all the schools. These regional gaps, then, formed the basis of our first curriculum development projects (explained below) which were funded over the course of the next four years.

THE RESULTING COMPETENCY-BASED
CHILD WELFARE CURRICULUM

Staff organized the final 1991 version of the competencies into six categories according to the task required and the topic under consideration.[5] The categories comprising the CalSWEC competencies for public child welfare MSW practice are: *Multicultural and Ethnic Sensitive Practice, Core Child Welfare Skills, Social Work Skills and Methods, Human Development and Behavior, Workplace Management, and Child Welfare Administration, Planning, and Evaluation.* The competency based approach was used to demonstrate that it

TABLE 3. The 1991 Top Three Competencies Lacking in Child Welfare Social Work Education by California Region*

Northern/Bay Region

1. Cultural understanding and use of supports.
2. Being able to deal with nonvoluntary and hostile clients.
3. Understanding the policy and legal basis for child welfare services and the goals of public social services.

Mountain Valley Region

1. Understanding cultural differences needed for assessment and practice.
2. Understanding policy and legal requirements for implementation.
3. Evaluation of abuse and neglect while understanding the trauma of separation.

Southern Region

1. Being able to deal with nonvoluntary and hostile clients.
2. Adapting the casework plan to a cultural perspective.
3. Interviewing in the home and in chaos and empowering families.

*Represents the consensus of the attendees at the first curriculum implementation conference, including faculty and practitioners.

was truly possible for schools of social work to integrate very specific field related knowledge and skills and yet provide a broad-based educational experience for students. It was expected that the competencies would change over time as at-risk groups comprising the service population change, as more knowledge is developed about what works, and as policy changes.

To further emphasize the importance of a guiding philosophical statement, the National Association of Public Child Welfare Administrators survey found that "The greatest barrier to collaboration between child welfare agencies and schools of social work is the absence of a common philosophy and a shared agenda between these two institutions" [NAPCWA, 1991: 3]. In response, staff included a statement of guiding principles in the list of competencies. Some important factors in the guiding statement for the competency-based curriculum should be stressed: This statement philosophically supports a wide diversity of life styles, including many definitions of family. It recognizes the state's right to intervene to protect children, while encouraging workers to make reasonable efforts to keep families together. It also supports the importance of delivering effective service based on empirically based procedures and literature. Critical thinking is encouraged. Finally, it acknowledges, above and beyond the professional definition of each individual competency section, the family's contribution to the definition of the child welfare situation.

Multicultural and Ethnic Sensitive Practice items received the most agreement from all concerned who felt that ethnically sensitive practice skills should be applied throughout the competency document and also be described in a special section so that these issues would be neither isolated nor underemphasized. This section presumes that the practitioner will go beyond the simple understanding of cultural differences: to apply social work techniques and knowledge to learn the values of the client family, contrast them with dominant values, and to effectively use that knowledge to foster culturally sensitive treatment plans. This knowledge must then be transferred to the student's field experience in order to build skills in cultural competency. Specifically this section includes essential knowledge, values, and skills for culturally competent child welfare practice with particular attention to the context of oppression and racism, the role of culture in an individual's well being, and an understanding of the diversity represented by the people of California.

Core Child Welfare Skills contains the assessment categories and specialized topics included in the field's categorization of child welfare services. Highlighted in this section are the various kinds of conflict that child welfare workers must be knowledgeable about to do their jobs: Spousal, substance, and institutional abuse in addition to the different kinds of child abuse. Here are competencies emphasizing the child welfare worker's role with the court system. This section also identifies the important target populations which seem to constitute most of the child welfare cases in California now: persons of color who are overrepresented in the child welfare system, low income families, single parent families, medically fragile children in foster care, and nontraditional families, including kinship foster care. It is in this section that specific competencies for knowledge about the legal basis for intervention and working with the legal dependency system are found. Finally, the child welfare worker's dual responsibility to the family as well as the child and the collaboration required to provide effective services are incorporated.

The third section, *Social Work Skills and Methods*, features skills that are core to direct practice social work education, combining these skills with specialized knowledge about families, adolescents and very young children. Interviewing hostile and nonvoluntary clients is acknowledged as a special skill. It highlights the differences from the usual casework methods of interviewing voluntary clients. There are competencies which address the student's ability to interview and adapt treatment plans to adverse conditions, such as home visiting and interviewing in chaotic environments, for example, interviewing family members outside courtrooms or teenagers at bus stops.

The core technique used in this section is case management. The conception of case management encompasses assessment and interviewing skills, self awareness, and critical thinking skills, so important in this field. Case management skills such as, making initial and ongoing risk assessments regarding child safety and family functioning, appropriate referrals for community resources, recommendations to the court about placement, working with community groups to support a family in reunification are emphasized in this field of practice. They also require the ability to work in interdisciplinary teams or at least work side by side with others concerned for child protection and permanency.

The child welfare worker must be well versed in the assessment, treatment, and support of caregivers who face mental health and/or substance abuse problems, especially since adult mental health and substance abuse problems, which often accompany severe cases of abuse and neglect, recur with varying levels of severity.

The section on *Human Development and Behavior* takes into account the effect of societal, structural, and environmental factors on the phenomenon of child abuse and neglect, adoptions, and placement. However, normal human development must be studied also to discern what differential effects child abuse, neglect, and family problems have on various members of the family at different times of their lives. This is important to treatment planning to design age level appropriate individual treatment plans for child welfare clients. Learning about the effects of developmental disabilities and special medical needs of children from substance abusing environments and those who have HIV is included here.

It is important to note that the focus is on child development and the effects of loss and separation on children and families. This is different from the required generalist MSW human behavior and social environment courses that teach human development across the life span. There has been much discussion about the development of the brains of young children, when most enter foster care, beyond the separation and attachment theory literature, and the need for quick intervention to protect brain development [Wolfe, 1991; Dawson et al., 1994; Silverman, 1996; Illig, 1998].

This knowledge has been pivotal in the development of social policy, namely the Adoption and Safe Families Act (P.L. 105-89), which emphasizes early permanency for children and deplores the effects of foster care drift on children. To the extent that the policy has created new opportunities for adoption of children who formerly would have languished too long in foster care, this policy has the effect of placing time lines on the services support system for any family referred for a child welfare issue. To the extent that the legal permanency fosters emotional permanency, this is good. For a worker to make the correct placement at the right time requires an extensive knowledge of child and family development. The social workers in this field have to know the difference because this is central to defining a successful outcome for a child and a family.

Workplace Management recognizes that the agency organizational culture and agency policy interpretation influences practice. In most social work programs, students either focus on direct or indirect skills. One consequence of this dichotomy is that direct service social workers may not comprehend the full range of influence an organization can have on the individual practitioner and his or her client and do not understand what options they have for dealing with organizations to get things done for their clients. In the field of child welfare, workers as team members, regularly encounter problems in interorganizational relationships with court systems, schools, hospitals, and other large traditional bureaucracies. They must be able to show their expertise to enhance their credibility and to accomplish their goals.

Workplace management emphasizes worker competence in dealing with distress. Workplace management includes the achievement of competence in recognizing the contribution of and involving the community in child welfare concerns. The experience of the CalSWEC collaborators is that providing opportunities for ongoing adult learning contributes to retention and protects against burnout for child welfare workers. It follows that this section includes concepts of self care, peer support, conflict resolution, use of supervision, safety, and other aspects of the organizational climate. With the focus on retention of professional social workers and recruitment, the field is recognizing that better-prepared workers in supportive organizations can provide services with better outcomes for families and children [Glisson & Hemmelgarn, 1998].

The last category, *Child Welfare Administration Planning and Evaluation*, was included as part of the graduate social work curriculum for all students, though it is recognized that not all direct practice students can have a management experience in the field. However, this section addresses the importance policy on practice, as well as the issue of including organizational behavior and the effects of organizational structure on direct practice. Some schools include their research sequence in this section as a demonstration that MSWs provide a unique expertise in the area of practice and program evaluation.

CURRICULUM MODIFICATION

The project coordinators led the effort to modify the curriculum competencies in 1996. By the time the curriculum was modified for the first time, the practitioners, who in 1991 had recommended that the schools not teach these advanced competencies, were ready to take responsibility for teaching them to students in the field and wanted classroom content about social work in the legal dependency system to complement those experiences. In that five years, due to resources focused on curriculum development and field placement enhancement, there were regular opportunities for students to participate in legal proceedings and write court reports. Agencies began to gain confidence that the students were focusing on their need for specialized training in child welfare.

In 2001, the second major modification of the curriculum will occur after a series of community focus groups conducted by the project coordinators at each school and a series of CalSWEC meetings with the project coordinators and the board. So far, the competency list has held up: Participants are updating, grouping and combining the competencies in ways that could not have happened in 1991 because they did not have experience with each others' institutional language. Participants in these focus groups include field instructors, child welfare workers and supervisors, former IV-E students, attorneys, administrators, foster parents, and former foster youth.

Preliminary analysis indicates that there will be fewer competencies and they will be organized according to first and second year MSW program. Through the years, as goals, services and populations shift, the understanding of what MSWs should know and be able to do will need to be revisited, revised, and upgraded. A postgraduate list that may give us a more thorough picture of our extended goals for the MSW child welfare practitioner in California through the two year postgraduate level would be important to start developing now.

Now that an extensive partnership of schools and agencies has agreed upon a competency-based child welfare curriculum, how well the curriculum will continue to be woven into the existing curricula at the (now)14 graduate schools of social work in California remains the work of the collaboration. In discussing implementation, it is important to remember that this list of competencies represents the minimum skill and knowledge expectations for the newly graduated MSW specializing in child welfare.

Title IV-E funding has been used here to develop new curricula in fields germane to child welfare, such as interprofessional collaboration, ethnic sensitive practice, and working with kinship foster families. Schools have held faculty development seminars for field instructors to learn how to apply the competencies in their settings. Some specialized child welfare courses have been developed, such as Working with Vulnerable Children (CSWE, 1999). Most of the integrative field seminars are focused on the transfer of learning between the classroom and the field.

EVALUATION AND INCENTIVES FOR CHANGE

It is important to see the competency-based curriculum as a work in progress, not as a rigid and eternal set of standards. The Center conducts an assessment, monitoring, and evaluation process to learn the effects of the competency-based curriculum in California. One of the criticisms of a competency-based approach to knowledge and skill building is that it is normatively generated. This is akin to the criticism of social work practice that it is "authority-based" or not easily amenable to change or open to the consideration of values that go beyond the limitations of existing policies and procedures [Gambrill, 2001]. Consequently social work practice does not reflect what is truly helpful for clients because it has not been empirically evaluated. That having been said, this particular model of collaboration, although it resulted in a consensus-based curriculum, set the conditions for creating empirically-based practice and curricula.

The next steps in the monitoring process consisted of evaluation of the curriculum: Is it being taught by the schools? After the stipend program had been in effect for one semester in May 1993, project coordinators at each of the 10 schools involved in the coalition took "snapshots" of the existing curricula. The first snapshots were baseline measures of the curricula before the development of specialized field seminars and the application of other curriculum development resources.

Currently, schools present a progress curriculum snapshot report each June. These snapshots indicate where the schools have refined and updated information regarding where the competencies are found (in the field or in the classroom) and when (in the first or second year of the graduate program). They also identify where resources are needed for curriculum development and instructional support. A second source of data, along with the snapshots, is focus group information from graduating students at each school, gathered to identify gaps and strengths in the curriculum. When students complete their work payback requirements, they are sent a survey designed to assess their intent to remain or leave child welfare and to investigate the organizational and educational implications of their experiences [Dickinson & Perry, 1998].

Several CalSWEC schools have developed their own evaluation instruments for measuring individual student competence using the competency-based curriculum, but the general feeling has been that the MSW program itself has sufficient measures (exams, field instructor evaluations, for example) that new ones are not necessary. This may or may not be the case: The purpose of measuring skill and knowledge in this particular field is to connect the learning with better outcomes for child welfare practice. The Center applies the knowledge gained from the snapshots, the student focus groups and the ongoing retention study to redirect resources for change. For example, to begin to make changes in the curricula, in 1993-4 members of the coalition proposed curriculum development awards that would enhance teaching of the competencies initially identified in the snapshot as absent or weak in the curricula or ranked in the 1991 regional groups as important but not adequately acquired. The awards produced several best practices curriculum workbooks and videotapes.[6]

The research and development committee of the board, consisting of county welfare directors and university deans and directors, garnered research questions from the practitioner community. Then, using these practitioner-based questions, requests for the schools of social work for applied research projects that would result in curricula that would be made available to all the schools. These projects resulted in a variety of empirically based curricula.[7] Although starting from a consensus model of curriculum competencies, the resources have been directed at creating more opportunities among the schools and agencies to develop empirically based curriculum for practice.

In addition, regional groups of schools and county agencies held faculty development institutes that included field supervisors and classroom faculty. In some instances, it was the first time a group of schools had collaborated on a presentation to the practitioner community. In others, although the group had collaborated before, the opportunity to provide specialized focus on child welfare issues had not previously occurred.

By comparing the state of the agency-university collaboration from the beginning of academic year 1992-1993 to the end of academic year 1994-1995, there have been positive changes. After only 3 years the curriculum snapshots from the schools showed an increase in the number and the kinds of opportunities for collaboration among the schools and the agencies for applied research and development of services.

Table 4 shows that there have been increases since 1992 in all categories of faculty agency collaboration, except one. There have not been any faculty who have taken leave to work at a public child welfare agency. However, more faculty are collaborating on applied research projects at the local county agencies and perhaps that is the structure that fits the skill of the faculty as well as the incentive system of the university, rather than taking a leave for practice experience alone.

CHALLENGES

Critics say that by preparing social workers for a specific field of practice, the foundation of social work education is compromised. Challenges for this and other projects like it include first demonstrating which skills and knowledge social workers bring to the child welfare arena and to show that with this better preparation, workers will produce better outcomes for disadvantaged children and families. Logical next steps would be to collaboratively develop recommendations for research on the relationship between professional educa-

TABLE 4. Numbers of Faculty Involved in Public Child Welfare In California

	1992-93	1993-94	1994-95
Serving on public child welfare committees	24	21	24
Serving on public child welfare agency commissions	15	15	7
On academic leave for work in public child welfare	0	0	0
Involved in the development of service pilots	19	23	26
Providing consultation for public child welfare agencies	28	26	54
Providing inservice training for public child welfare employees	37	23	58
Conducting collaborative research with public child welfare agencies	28	25	48

September 18, 1995

tion and worker retention as well as on outcomes for families and children who are served by professional social workers.

The use of competencies holds promise in several areas. First, if applied systematically and examined in terms of what is required on the job, competencies could be used to help agencies differentially assign cases to differently educated levels of social workers. With a competency-based curriculum specially designed for this work, the connection between agency-based on the job training and professional social work education can be strengthened. By encouraging on the job training, support is given to the public child welfare agency as a learning organization. The agencies will be able to "grow their own" MSWs by recruiting them early in their careers and connecting training and educational opportunities to incentives for promotion and recognition

The buy-in process needs to be refreshed periodically. When new members of the collaboration join the board, a complete orientation is crucial, so that they can understand and support the program. New partners from other disciplines, such as school social work and mental health should be encouraged to participate and to develop shared field experiences for students rather than competing for them. The point, after all, is to start where the families' needs are.

CONCLUSION:
INTERDEPENDENT COMPONENTS OF THE MODEL
REINFORCE EACH OTHER

Although this project and the means for evaluating it have limitations, it has been successful in creating opportunities for agency-university partnerships and for increasing professional development opportunities for child welfare workers. Among its limitations are first, that it has not systematically established that better outcomes for children and families result from specially trained MSWs. Secondly, although CalSWEC has an eight year track record and a fair amount of success with agency-university collaborations, we still do not know how well these connections will be sustained during a period in which there are shortages of many different kinds of social workers or changes in public policy about IV-E funding. Third, our means for evaluating graduate outcomes need to be strengthened; that is we need to better operationalize the competencies and be able to say clearly what a specially trained IV-E MSW knows and is able to do upon graduation.

Public policy has established a focus on permanency and safety for children, to break the cycle of multiple foster homes for dependent children. These objectives require child welfare departments to radically alter the scope and focus of services. In addition, as noted above, members of ethnic, racial, and cultural minority groups constitute an increasing portion of the clientele of the child welfare system. This condition requires increased recruitment of minority workers and the mastery by all workers of culturally competent practice. Besides mastering new intervention modes, students who enter public social welfare practice in the next few years must have the leadership and organizational skills to play significant roles in improving the structure and design of agencies and service programs.

To enhance collaboration the opportunity for exchange must be present: Use of the competency-based curriculum, in this case, was and is the key. For a collaborative partnership to be mutually beneficial to families, schools, and agencies, common definitions of the problems families and children face must be agreed upon, social workers must have adequate opportunities to learn about them, and research must be directed toward the alleviation of the negative human conditions that cause them.

NOTES

1. Center operations are funded by a combination of Title IV-E federal funding through the Department of Health and Human Services and private foundation funds. A three year grant from the Ford Foundation was extended to five years and supplemented by the Haas, Walter S. Johnson, Lurie, San Francisco, Santa Clara, Stuart, van Loben Sels, and Zellerbach funds. The authors would like to thank the Federal Regional Office of the Administration for Children, Youth and Family, and the Department of Social Services, State of California for their support of graduate child welfare social work education through Title IV-E funds. Ms. Lisa C. Tracy contributed to the development of this report.

2. The actual California Competency-Based Child Welfare Curriculum for gradu ate social work education is not included here but is available to interested readers on the CalSWEC Web page: (http://calswec.berkeley.edu).

3. As of fall, 2001, there were 14 California graduate schools of social work involved with the CalSWEC program.

4. The first additional source was a list of in-service training competencies developed for the State of California Emergency Response Training Project at California State University at Fresno by Wynn Tabbert, Peggy Sullivan and Robert Whittaker (1988), entitled, *An empirical validation of competencies required for child protective services practice*. The second was a list of fieldwork competencies developed at Cal State Long Beach under the direction of Janet Black, Teri Hughes, and Jeanne Crose, entitled, *Fundamental and Specialized Child Welfare Competencies*, plus handouts, from a workshop entitled, *Building Child Welfare Practitioners*, Anaheim, CA, October 5, 1990.

5. *The Statement of Principles and the Curriculum Competencies for Public Child Welfare Practice* in California can be obtained from the CalSWEC web site, address previously noted.

6. For example: two involved ethnic sensitive practice, one developed a workbook for specialized child welfare skills, one integrated management skills and knowledge into direct practice, one involved the effect of substance abuse on child welfare, and one navigated through the hazardous (for social workers) child welfare legal system. These can be obtained through the CalSWEC library accessed through the CalSWEC website.

7. For example, in 1997-1998 Academic Year, the following projects were funded: *The Effects of Computerization on Public Child Welfare Practice* Dale Weaver, CSU, Long Beach; David Cherin, USC. Duncan Lindsey, UCLA.
Choices: The Effectiveness of Court Mandated Intervention versus Voluntary Services in Child Protective Services. Loring Jones, San Diego State University.
Children's Experiences of Out-of-Home Care: Elements of a Successful Foster Care System. Jill Duerr Berrick and Barbara Needell, UC Berkeley.

BIBLIOGRAPHY

Albers, E.C., Reilly, T., & Rittner, B. (1993) Children in foster care: Possible factors affecting permanency planning. *Child and Adolescent Social Work Journal*, 10 (4): 329-341.

Berube, M., Director of Editorial Operations. (1985) *The American Heritage Dictionary*. Boston, MA: Houghton-Mifflin.

Blome, W. Whiting (1998) What is the effect of litigation on children and families in the child welfare system?: A review of the literature and litigation documents. (Unpublished paper.)

Blome, W. Whiting (1996) Reasonable efforts, unreasonable effects: A retrospective analysis of the 'reasonable efforts' clause in the Adoption Assistance and Child Welfare Act of 1980. *Journal of Sociology and Social Welfare.* XXIII (3): 133–150.

Booz-Allen and Hamilton, Inc. (1987, January) *The Maryland social work services job analysis and personnel qualifications study.* Baltimore, MD: Maryland Department of Human Resources.

California Welfare Directors' Association. (1986) Informal study done by M. Buck, president of CWDA. Numbers provided to B. Grossman. Sacramento, CA: CWDA..

Cheung, K., Stevenson, K. M., and Leung, P. (1991) Competency-based evaluation of case-management skills in child sexual abuse intervention *Child Welfare,* LXX(4): 425-436.

Child Welfare League of America. (1990). *Florida recruitment and retention study.* Washington, DC: Author.

Child Welfare and AIDS Project (1991) *Child welfare protocols for children with HIV infection: Guidelines for development and evaluation.* Berkeley, CA: University of California, School of Social Welfare, Child Welfare and AIDS Project.

Choi, J. (1992) Attributes of professions and their implication to the social work profession experiencing the growth of private practice. Unpublished paper. Berkeley, CA: School of Social Welfare, University of California at Berkeley.

Council on Social Work Education. (1994) Curriculum policy for the master's degree programs in social work education. In *CSWE handbook of accreditation standards and procedures* (pp.134-144). Alexandria, VA: Council on Social Work Education.

Dawson, G.; Hessl, D.; Frey, K. (1994) Social influences on early developing biological and behavioral systems related to risk for affective disorder. *Developmental Psychopathology.* 6: 759-779.

Delbeq, A.; Van den Ven, A. H.; and Gustafson, D. H. (1975) *Group techniques for program planning: A guide to nominal group and Delphi processes.* Glenwood, Il: Scott, Foresman and Company.

Dickinson, N. & Perry, R.E. (1998) *Why do MSWs stay in public child welfare?: Organizational and training implications of a retention study.* Presentation to the 11th National Conference of the National Staff Development and Training Association. New Orleans, Louisiana. December 8, 1998.

Freisen, B. J. (1989) Child mental health training in schools of social work: A national survey. In Abramczyk, L. W. *Social work education for working with seriously emotionally disturbed children and adolescents.* [S.l.]: National Association of Deans and Directors of Schools of Social Work.

Gambrill, E. (2001) Social work: An authority-based profession. *Research on Social Work Practice.* 11(2): 166–187.

Gambrill, E. (1983) *Casework: A competency based approach.* Englewood Cliffs, N.J.: Prentice-Hall.

Grossman, B., Laughlin, S., & Specht, H. (1992) Building the commitment of social work education to publicly supported social services: The California model. In

Briar, K.H., Hansen, V. H., and Harris, N., eds. *New partnerships: Proceedings from the national public child welfare training symposium.* Miami, FL: Florida International University.

Harris, N.; Kirk, R. S.; & Besharov, D. (1993) *State child welfare agency staff survey report.* Washington, DC: National Child Welfare Leadership Center, Inc.

Helfgott, K. P. (1991) *Staffing the child welfare agency: Recruitment and retention.* Washington, DC: Child Welfare League of America.

Hughes, R. C. and Rycus, J. S. (1989) *Target: Competent staff.* Washington D.C. and Columbus, OH: Child Welfare League of America and the Institute of Human Services.

Illig, D. C. (1998) *Birth to Kindergarten: The Importance of the Early Years.* Sacramento, CA: California Research Bureau.

Institute for Human Services. (1987, September 1) Individual training needs assessment for child welfare caseworkers. Columbus, OH: Author.

Kravitz, S. (1992) Professional social work education and public child welfare. In Briar, K. H., Hansen, V. H., and Harris, N., eds. *New partnerships: Proceedings from the national public child welfare training symposium.* Miami, FL: Florida International University.

Lauffer, A. (1984) *Strategic marketing for not-for-profit organizations.* New York, NY: Free Press.

Lauderdale, M., Grinnell, R. and McMurtry, S. (1980, November) Child welfare curricula in schools of social work: A national survey. *Child Welfare,* LIX(9): 531-541.

LeCroy, C. W. (1990, October 12) A model curriculum for training social workers for practice with severely emotionally disturbed children and adolescents. Paper presented at NIMH Conference on Child and Adolescent Mental Health, Berkeley, CA.

Lieberman, A. A., Hornsby, H. & Russell, M. (1988). Analyzing the educational backgrounds and work experiences of child welfare personnel: a national study. *Social Work,* 33(6): 485-89.

Mace, J.P. (2000) Social work jobs going unfilled in California. *NASW News.* September.

Maine Child Welfare Training Institute (1991) A new paradigm for competency-based training. Draft report. Portland, ME: University of Southern Maine.

National Association of Public Child Welfare Administrators (1991) *Public child welfare agencies and schools of social work: The current status of collaboration.* Washington, D.C.: Author.

National Association of Social Workers (1989a, November) *NASW California News.* Sacramento, CA: Author.

National Association of Social Workers (1989b) *The staffing crisis in child welfare: Report from a colloquium.* Silver Spring, MD: Author.

Negron-Velasquez, G; Clark, S.; & Brown, E. (1995) *The CalSWEC Workforce Study.* Berkeley, CA: CalSWEC, University of California, Berkeley.

Olsen, L. & Holmes, W.M. (1982). Educating child welfare workers: the effects of professional training on service delivery. *Journal of Education for Social Work,* 18(1): 94-102.

Patterson, K. (2000) *Redesigning Utah's child welfare system*. Presentation to the New Century Child Welfare and Family Support National Conference. Snowbird, UT. September, 2000.

Pecora, P. et al. (1990) *National CPS competency-based training project: Final report and list of available training materials*. Salt Lake City, UT: Graduate School of Social Work University of Utah.

Perry, R.; Limb, G.; & Clark, S.; (1998) *Workforce Study of California's Public Child Welfare Workers*. Berkeley: California Social Work Education Center, University of California, Berkeley, CA.

Russell, M. (1987). *National study of public child welfare job requirements*. Portland, ME: University of Southern Maine, National Resource Center for Management and Administration.

Samantrai, K. (1990, September, October, November,December) MSWs in public welfare: Why do they stay, and why do they leave? Parts 1-4. *NASW California News*. Sacramento, CA: National Association of Social Workers, California chapter.

Samantrai, K. (1992, September) "Factors in the decision to leave: Retaining MSWs in public child welfare" *Social Work* 37(6).

Schneiderman, L., Cohen, J.F., Waldinger, G., and Furman, W. (1990) *Social work practitioners panels: Connecting social work practice to social policy*. Los Angeles, CA: University of California at Los Angeles, School of Social Welfare, Center for Child and Family Policy Studies.

Shyne, A.W. & Schroeder, A.G. (1978) *National study of social services to children and their families*. Prepared for National Center for Child Advocacy, U.S. Children's Bureau, DHEW. Rockville, MD: Westat, Inc.

Silverman, A.; Reinherz, H.Z.; Glaclonia, R.M. (1996) The long term sequelae of child and adolescent abuse: A longitudinal community study. *Child Abuse and Neglect*. 20: 709-723.

Simmons, M. (1990) Informal study done by the director of Tulare County (California) Public Social Services Department. Numbers provided to B. Grossman.

Sokal, K. and Ramler, M. (1991) *Children and families and HIV: A training curriculum for social service and health providers*. Berkeley, CA: University of California, School of Social Welfare, Child Welfare and AIDS Project.

Tabbert, W. and Sullivan, P. (1988) *An empirical validation of competencies required for child protective services practice*. Draft report. California State University, Fresno, CA: Author.

Tatara, T. (1991) *Characteristics of children in substitute care: A statistical summary of the VCIS national child welfare data base: Based on FY 87 data*. Voluntary Cooperative Information System. Washington D.C: American Public Welfare Association.

Wertkin, R. and Hansen, K. (1991, March) Linking social education to public welfare: Let's get specific. Paper presented at the Annual Program Meeting of the Council on Social Work Education, New Orleans, LA.

Wiltse, K. (1981) *Education and training for child welfare practice: The search for a better fit.* Mimeo. The University of California at Berkeley: Author.

Wolfe, D.A. McGee, R. (1991) Assessment of emotional status among maltreated children. In Starr, R. & Wolfe, D., eds. *The Effects of Child Abuse and Neglect: Issues and Research.* New York, N.Y.: Guilford Press; pp. 257-277.

Wolfe, L.C., ed., (1989) *Collaboration for competency: Examining social work curriculum in the perspective of current practice with children and families.* Lexington, KY: The University of Kentucky, College of Social Work.

Wong, J. (February 9, 2001) Hearing on the Shortage of Social Workers in California. Presentation to Hon. Dion Aroner, Assemblywoman & Chair of the Human Services Committee of the California State Assembly.

Design Teams as Learning Systems for Complex Systems Change: Evaluation Data and Implications for Higher Education

Hal A. Lawson
Dawn Anderson-Butcher
Nancy Petersen
Carenlee Barkdull

SUMMARY. Systems change in child welfare and cross-systems change involving other service sectors are needed in response to two developments: (1) New policy mandates (e.g., TANF, ASFA) and (2) Research on the co-occurring and interlocking needs of many child welfare families.

A four-state initiative was structured in response to these needs. Collaborative learning and action research groups called *design teams* were structured to identify competencies and to develop new service delivery systems. Faculty facilitators representing social work education programs were assigned to these teams and charged with their development and evaluation. Facilitators served as linkage agents for university-commu-

Hal A. Lawson is affiliated with The University at Albany, SUNY.
Dawn Anderson-Butcher is affiliated with The Ohio State University.
Nancy Petersen is affiliated with The University of Nevada-Reno.
Carenlee Barkdull is affiliated with The University of Utah.

[Haworth co-indexing entry note]: "Design Teams as Learning Systems for Complex Systems Change: Evaluation Data and Implications for Higher Education." Lawson, Hal A. et al. Co-published simultaneously in *Journal of Human Behavior in the Social Environment* (The Haworth Social Work Practice Press, an imprint of The Haworth Press, Inc.) Vol. 7, No. 1/2, 2003, pp. 159-179; and: *Charting the Impacts of University-Child Welfare Collaboration* (ed: Katharine Briar-Lawson, and Joan Levy Zlotnik) The Haworth Social Work Practice Press, an imprint of The Haworth Press, Inc., 2003, pp. 159-179. Single or multiple copies of this article are available for a fee from The Haworth Document Delivery Service [1-800-HAWORTH, 9:00 a.m. - 5:00 p.m. (EST). E-mail address: getinfo@haworthpressinc.com].

nity-state agency partnerships, and they promoted curriculum change.

These study reports two sets of findings related to these design teams: (1) Findings from semi-structured interviews of design team members; and (2) Findings from the participatory action research completed by two faculty facilitators. Key themes related to design team processes are presented. Drawing on these emergent themes, components that help explain effective design team processes are identified. Selected implications for social work education programs and faculty also are identified *[Article copies available for a fee from The Haworth Document Delivery Service: 1-800-HAWORTH. E-mail address: <getinfo@haworthpressinc.com> Website: <http://www.HaworthPress.com> © 2003 by The Haworth Press, Inc. All rights reserved.]*

KEYWORDS. Collaborative learning, action research, systems change

"We didn't have the kind of service delivery system we needed. *We had to design it first.* Then we could plan and deliver our training" (Abernathy, 2000, emphasis added). This concise statement was provided by a former client called *a family expert,* and it introduces a four-state child welfare initiative. This initiative was structured to improve child welfare practice, social work education programs, and university-agency-community partnerships. It promoted practice innovations, systems change, and cross-systems change.

Design teams were formed in four states (Colorado, Utah, Nevada, and New Mexico). These design teams consisted of family experts (i.e., former and current service recipients), university faculty facilitators, and professionals from child welfare and other service systems. These teams comprised new learning and development systems. They used participatory action research and collaborative action research to design new collaborative practices involving interprofessional, family-centered, and community collaboration (Anderson-Butcher, Lawson, & Barkdull, in press; Lawson & Barkdull, 2001; Lawson, Petersen, & Briar-Lawson, 2001). In brief, these design teams engaged in collaborative learning. As they learned, they developed new practice innovations, while identifying competencies needed for these innovations.

In addition, these teams were vehicles for practice research and faculty development. For example, teams generated new knowledge and understanding about collaborative practices. They helped faculty facilitators appreciate the differences between learning systems and training systems (Lawson, 2000), both in community settings and in social work education programs. Many such details of the design team model, including relevant theory and evaluation data, must be omitted from this publication because of space constraints. Readers interested in design teams should consult other publications (e.g., Anderson-Butcher, Lawson, & Barkdull, in press; Lawson, 2000a; Lawson & Barkdull, 2001; Lawson, Petersen, & Briar-Lawson, 2001).

Here, the analysis focuses on the roles and responsibilities of faculty facilitators, some of the mechanics of the design team process (including barriers and enabling factors), and a few of the implications for higher education in general and social work education in particular. Where faculty facilitators are concerned, two kinds of evaluation data are featured. Data about design team processes and the faculty facilitators, gathered by an external evaluator (Anderson-Butcher), are presented. Then data derived from the participatory action research completed by two faculty facilitators (Petersen and Barkdull) are presented. Finally, implications for social work education programs are identified.

EVALUATING THE DESIGN TEAM PROCESS AND THE WORK OF FACULTY FACILITATORS

The design team evaluation included two data sets, which are presented next. The first set derives from interviews of design team members. The second derives from the participatory action research of two faculty facilitators.

An external evaluator (Anderson-Butcher) conducted qualitative interviews with 22 long-standing design team members in order to gain an in-depth understanding about the design team experience and process. Nine of the members interviewed were university-based facilitators; six were family experts; three were middle managers in child welfare; two were state child welfare administrators; and, two were front-line professionals from other service systems. Sixteen were female; six were male.

Nine open-ended questions guided the interview. Examplary questions include: (1) What do you believe have been the major accomplishments of the design team(s)? (2) Have you encountered barriers; and if so, what are they and how did you or others involved deal with them? (3) What have you learned as a result of your involvement? (4) What have been some of the high points and low points related to your involvement? And, (7) Can you share any lessons learned from the experience? Each interview lasted approximately 40 minutes. The researcher used probes, as needed, throughout the interview process. She took notes were taken throughout the interviews and later transcribed them.

The researcher derived direct quotes from each interview. Each quote represented single items or themes (see Miles & Huberman, 1994). The raw data were then coded into classification schemes using inductive techniques (Patton,

1990). Consensus validation was established with a peer reviewer who was familiar with the data (Lincoln & Guba, 1985). The peer reviewer correctly coded 87% of the raw data quotes, indicating moderate to high validity. When discrepancies were found, the researcher and the peer reviewer would together re-cluster the themes, establishing consistency between them and enhancing the validity of the classification.

Themes related to design team implementation and resultant outcomes emerged from the data. Only those themes related to Design Team implementation are presented in this article; outcomes associated with design teams are reported in Anderson-Butcher, Lawson, and Barkdull (in press).

Where design team implementation is concerned, three higher order themes emerged from the interview data. These themes included issues related to implementation, leadership, and barriers. Tables 1, 2, and 3 describe the themes and the number of Design Team members interviewed that mentioned the theme. Parentheses indicate the frequency of responses mentioned by all participants. In addition, A brief overview is provided here.

The most common themes mentioned by participants were related to Design Team member recruitment. The most common theme mentioned was discussed by 82% of the participants. They noted how there needed to be the recruitment of the "right people," including people who are in administrative roles with power, those with informal power, and those that are change agents that "make things happen."

Participants also noted that recruitment should focus on fitting the agendas of people, agencies, and current policies. Each theme was mentioned by 77%, 55%, and 82% of the people interviewed, respectively.

Furthermore, 32% of the people discussed issues related to the need to court the agencies or people that are resistant; whereas over 26% discussed the importance of the facilitators in relying on their past relationships for recruitment. The facilitators needed (1) the skills to bring people together; and (2) the passion to keep things moving. For instance, 55% noted the importance of having a person on the Design Team (i.e., the facilitator) who would do the legwork, follow-up and coordinate efforts; whereas 32% discussed the facilitator's persistence and energy.

The second major theme that emerged from the interviews was related to group dynamics within the Design Teams. 32% noted that the Design Teams had to be a place that set the stage for equality. This ensured that family experts felt "safe" discussing their past experiences, front-line professionals felt "comfortable" talking about issues in front of administrators, and people from different "professions" did not feel threatened by others unlike them. Facilitators had a direct role in making this happen. For instances, 55% of participants noted that facilitators needed to create a safe environment for people. In other words,

TABLE 1. Content Analyses Examining Design Team "How To's."

Theme	Total	Examplary Quotes
1. FIT CURRENT AGENDAS		
• . . . of agency involved.	17(43)	"(Agency) was already looking at how to provide services that were family-centered. (Each agency got) to talk about what is new within their agency, helped get attendees there. They were telling others what they were doing."
• . . . of people involved.	14(19)	"I am interested in things that are community oriented, that's my background. DT resonated with my goals."
• . . . of the law or policy.	6(7)	"There has been a concern about vulnerable families due to welfare reform and time limits, vulnerable now are much more vulnerable."
2. Get the power people there.	18(45)	"Buy-in from the administration is essential to go anywhere;" "(got) change agents there;" "can't just be anyone, needs to be big people."
3. Set stage for equality.	6(8)	"Modeled good communication styles; she always gives everyone a voice and that is what the grant was about."
4. Court groups/people that are resistant or hesitant.	7(7)	"Need to intervene with each person... .Maybe pull them aside and have them think about the bigger plan;" "I need to go back and make rounds, visit one to one these people."
5. Include players from the beginning.	2(3)	"We should write the grant with agencies involved from the start, also start top down."
6. Listen to the group about what works for them.	3(3)	"Let communities choose days and times."
7. Recruit participants.	6(10)	"(The facilitator) knew the players, and talked them into coming;" "Rounded up usual suspects."
8. Provide incentives.	5(11)	"It is the cheapest CEUs in town; ". . .pay FE, measure of respect. I am worth that;" "Snacks and liquids at no charge . . . to get people there."
9. Have someone to do the leg-work.	12(16)	"Need to do the leg work. Hand holding;" "Need the man power to coordinate the efforts."
10. Power in numbers.	3(3)	"What you need to do is outnumber them. This works."
11. Have university involved.	3(4)	"Third party from the University, the neutrality is helpful."
12. Have boosters and things to keep people involved.	1(3)	"We should give homework;" "Create steering committee sooner."
13. Have support to debrief.	2(4)	"We need immediate support, too. The processing afterwards is important."

Note: Totals provide information about the frequency and intensity of each theme. The first number indicates the total number of study participants that mentioned the theme. The number in parentheses indicates the number of times those subjects discussed the theme.

TABLE 2. Content Analyses Examining Themes Related to Leadership of Design Teams

Theme	Total	Example Item
SKILL AND ABILITY		
• Ability to bring people together.	7(8)	"Just getting people to table to talk, to connect"
• Ability to get people to buy-in.	3(3)	"I had to go . . . (the facilitator) is well known and respected."
• Group facilitation skills.	3(4)	"Need to shape and intervene, good facilitation skills are needed."
• Ability to get people to take ownership of the process.	10(32)	"I needed to let them take ownership in things: there were times when I knew what they wanted to do wouldn't work, but I couldn't tell them, it would backfire."
• Nurtures a safe environment to work together.	12(25)	"Gave people arena, safe place to cooperate and get along."
PERSONAL ATTRIBUTES		
• Leader's persistence and energy.	7(9)	"I was very impressed with (the leaders') pushing."
• Treats you like family, mentor, supportive"	4(6)	"They made us part of their family. So open and genuine."
• Keeps ego out of the way.	2(2)	"I love the way (the facilitator) is doing it, gets ego out of the way.
• Leader is open, flexible and receptive.	2(3)	"'If you can think of a better way, let's try it' is his philosophy."
• Leader has patience.	1(3)	"Being okay with setbacks is something I have learned. I learned patience, not believing that I am responsible for everything."
• People with vision	1(1)	"Visionaries need task people to do their work, put their vision into practice."

Note: Totals provide information about the frequency and intensity of each theme. The first number indicates the total number of study participants that mentioned the theme. The number in parentheses indicates the number of times those subjects discussed the theme.

facilitators needed to know how and have skills in making Design Team members feel comfortable. Having this "safe place" was essential for the creation of ownership with the Design Team process. 45% of participants interviewed noted that it was vital to get Design Team members to take "ownership" of the process.

The final theme involved barriers related to the Design Team process. Any time a large group of people is brought together in a collaborative way, there are struggles and tensions. Many of these struggles were mentioned as deterrents to the Design Team process. For instance, 36% discussed barriers related

TABLE 3. Content Analyses Examining Barriers Related to the Design Team Process.

Theme	Total
1. DESIGN TEAM IMPLEMENTATION CONCERNS	
A. *Leadership issues.*	
• Funding streams to support initiatives are missing.	12(22)
• There are unclear expectations.	8(18)
• There was miscommunication.	8(22)
• Leadership of DT is ineffective.	1(1)
• Lack of guidance.	1(1)
B. *Learning systems concerns.*	
• There are challenges related to evaluation.	15(34)
• Difficult to balance the process and task foci.	14(28)
• Ambiguous process.	4(6)
C. *Negative feelings resulted.*	
• Feelings of disappointment.	11(21)
• There are feelings of isolation and abandonment.	7(20)
• Negative feelings resulted.	3(6)
D. *Hard to get family experts there.*	
• Hard to get and support family experts.	3(8)
2. ISSUES WITH PEOPLE:	
A. *Some people just don't get it.*	
• People don't get along, in general.	10(20)
• People don't change.	7(7)
• People are apathetic.	3(6)
• People think they are doing it and they aren't.	4(5)
• People are fearful of process.	2(3)
B. *People have practice theories that aren't family centered.*	
• People don't respect family experts	8(15)
• People believe professionals knows best/silo	5(11)
• Competitiveness between people and sites.	1(3)
C. *People aren't there and they need to be.*	
• Don't have buy-in from top level administrators and people with power.	9(11)
• People and agencies need to be there and aren't.	4(8)

TABLE 3 (continued)

Theme	Total
3. AGENCY AND SYSTEMS BARRIERS	
A. *Agency norms.*	
• Agencies have philosophical frameworks that don't fit with the Design Team.	6(9)
• "Projectitus" within agencies.	
B. *System Barriers*	
• System barriers with bureaucracy.	12(26)
• System barriers with university.	7(11)
C. *Staff Concerns*	
• Time constraints.	14(22)
• Staff turnover.	7(15)
• Dropout/Attrition.	7(14)
• Workers have too much workload; agencies are understaffed.	3(5)
4. COMMUNITY/CONTEXT ISSUES	
• Contextual circumstances provide challenges.	13(30)
• The community isn't ready for this type of initiative.	4(8)
• Distance.	3(6)

Note: Totals provide information about the frequency and intensity of each theme. The first number indicates the total number of study participants that mentioned the theme. The number in parentheses indicates the number of times those subjects discussed the theme.

to unclear expectations; 36% described issues with miscommunication; whereas 50% noted that they experienced feelings of disappointment within the process. 45% mentioned that people just don't get along.

Many of the people interviewed discussed concerns about the non-directive, process-oriented and the "non-training-like nature" of the design team process. More specifically, 63% mentioned barriers with balancing processes and tasks; 36% said that some team members did not respect family experts; and 60% discussed struggles with making the design team process fit with local and contextual needs. 55% mentioned that oftentimes system barriers were hard to break down, especially those related to top-down, professional-knows-best perspectives. Finally, 68% discussed challenges related to evaluating non-structured, process-oriented learning systems.

For example, participants noted that some people didn't understand what the Design Team was about (45% mentioned), and others had belief systems that were antithetical to what the design team promotes (36% mentioned). Furthermore, 41% suggested that supervisors and managers, people in power, needed to be included on the design teams; and that teams were less effective because they were not included.

Respondents identified two other barriers. Time required for participation was the first. Specifically, 64% of the people interviewed identified time-related barriers that limit their participation in both learning and training initiatives. The other common barrier was mentioned by 55% of those interviewed. With the impending termination of the grants that supported this work, respondents expressed concern about future funding support for the design teams of the future.

PARTICIPATORY ACTION RESEARCH BY TWO FACULTY FACILITATORS

Two faculty facilitators (Barkdull and Petersen) completed participatory action research with Lawson. Five basic questions structured this research.

- What technical skills did you need?
- What technical skills did you acquire?
- What did you learn about the design team process and your role as a facilitator?
- What did you learn about yourself? Did you experience a change in your identity and commitments, your orientations toward learning, or both?
- What are the implications for university faculty and university curricula?

Nancy Petersen's Participatory Action Research

Technical Skills Needed and Acquired: When I began as the facilitator of the design team in Reno, I had served for almost eight years as the statewide training coordinator for the university-agency partnership between the School of Social Work, University of Nevada-Reno, and the state and county child welfare agencies. In this position at the university, I developed skills in training, curriculum development, adult learning, and group facilitation. I also had a good knowledge of the overall social service delivery system, its relationship to the child welfare system, and the individual service providers in these systems. As a result of these personal contacts and relationships, I was able to identify key participants fairly easily and obtain their agreement to participate in this project.

My training coordinator experiences were very helpful for many aspects of the design team process. I was able to apply some of my group facilitation knowledge to the structuring of the initial experiential exercises and group interactions for the design team. My curriculum development experience helped in pulling together the team's learning into the final training curriculum. I also drew upon my skills in organization and conceptualization as I pulled together complicated information and identified key points and themes from our discussions. My writing skills, which were already strong, flourished as I produced detailed minutes and memos that tried to capture the highlights as well as the details of our learning. (In hindsight, this written record turned out to be extremely valuable in the group's process. For example, when the team was feeling unsure of what it was accomplishing and where it was going, the written record enabled it to recognize and build on its past discussions, therefore creating a critical sense of achievement and providing the foundation for continuing progress.)

I also realized fairly early on that I would need additional skills in-group process in order to provide a better balance between content and process. It was far too easy to become involved in one side of an issue and lose my more objective facilitator perspective. I also needed to develop skills in collaboration, so that I could help structure the process in a way that would encourage the team members to collaborate among themselves and develop their ownership of the team. These skills were important to help me serve in the role of facilitator and record keeper rather than "the boss." The turf issues that are so evident in our service delivery systems are equally evident in the design team process and then in the facilitator's role itself. I needed to consciously continue to expand my skills and develop ways to involve people in all aspects of the process instead of trying to do it all myself.

Knowledge and understanding about the design team process and its facilitation. The design team process was exciting, challenging, absorbing, and also anxiety provoking, as it felt that we were "building the plane while flying it." Team members often commented to me that they weren't sure where we were going and what we were accomplishing. However, they also kept coming back because of the process, the relationships, and the sense that they were learning new ideas and values that truly challenged and reinvigorated their practice.

So, a fundamental aspect of my own learning about the design team experience was the critical importance of recognizing both process and content. Process is key in the development of relationships and open communication between design team members. Process is also very important because, fundamentally, a design team is more of a learning system than a training system. A design team involves mutual learning and teaching, which are both dependent on process.

Interestingly enough, to go one last step, the process actually became the foundation of the content of the training curriculum developed by the design team in Reno. From our experience in the design team, we had a renewed understanding and respect for the importance of relationship and process in the provision of *all* services. The new demands of our increasingly complicated and changing service delivery systems are characterized by more widespread and extensive collaborative efforts between professionals and families. The fundamental belief in relationship, which involves listening and respecting and avoiding judgment and then listening some more, is one that any service provider needs to ultimately "get," in order to be as effective in their practice with others as they can be.

However, there is also a need for a group to feel that it is developing specific (more traditional, if you will) content, or products that the group can point to as accomplishments and results. Content in this context includes such items as the development of competencies, that is, the identification of specific knowledge, skills, and awareness needed to accomplish a practice goal. It can also include the identification and design of specific policies that support a practice goal or the development of a specific training curriculum that addresses specific practice issues.

In addition to the dynamic tension between process and content, I also struggled with the tension between "being in control" and "letting it happen." My prior experience in training and my expertise as a trainer with knowledge to impart sometimes conflicted with the idea of the design team as a self-generating learning system that is dependent on its process for the mutual learning between members. In addition, the external expectations from the grant in the form of deliverables and the internal need of the team to actually produce a product made it even more tempting to be in charge in order to speed up the process.

I also learned how important– and difficult–it can be to establish a group mission for the team that everyone understands. And I finally learned that it requires the team to structure and take charge of its mutual learning and development, assuming joint responsibility and accountability. I spent considerable energy, with increasing frustration, trying to identify for the group WHAT we were trying to learn from one another. Was it agency process, goals and constraints? Was it client process, issues, strengths and needs? Was it our barriers to service? Was it client barriers to service? Were we looking at process or outcomes? What are the important components for collaboration? It was finally necessary for the team to go through its own discussion to discover for itself where it wanted to focus its attention, how to put this complex mix of ideas together, and what the team mission should be.

As a facilitator, there were always times when the team seemed to be more productive or on track than other times. When the process didn't seem to be accomplishing the mutual learning goal that the group was aiming for, it was helpful to try and ascertain whether it was a problem with the specific activity or whether it could be viewed as a broader issue reflecting the service delivery system itself. For example, in trying to learn from one another about the different expertise of the team members, it was difficult to find the best format to facilitate this learning. Formal presentations seemed to be too boring or too global or too detailed but more casual discussions seemed to leave out important information. We tried to ascertain if the problem seemed to be the activity itself and figure out a better way to get the information, perhaps with clearer expectations of what was to be taught.

Sometimes it seemed that the real problem and the related difficulties were representative of broader system issues. For example, some professionals think narrowly and concretely about their own systems, and others were reflecting the realities of turf issues, agency cultures, or comfort levels of sharing. When these issues arose, we tried to address them. The Reno design team never did figure out a clear answer to these questions. However, the team's discussion of these dynamics can be a very productive process for a team, and it can lead to important learning and growth.

Finally, I learned that being the facilitator of a learning system requires a greater time commitment than usually demanded by conventional training preparation. A facilitator must spend considerable time planning, reflecting, writing, calling people, and attending meetings between the big meetings. It is also extremely important to stay in touch with the family experts to keep them involved as much as possible. For some facilitators, this could be a very frustrating process as it requires a facilitator to rely on others, work on the collaborative processes, and pull information from many different sources. But it is important to realize that, while the process may be less efficient in terms of traditional product production, the resulting commitment, system learning, and real system change make the time involved well worth the effort.

What I learned about myself. To put it most simply, I found that being the facilitator of a design team was a life-changing experience. I gained new confidence in my existing abilities, expanded my skills into new areas, became much more active in my own learning process, and became much more willing to take risks. In my job at the university, I volunteered for some interdepartmental projects in the college, which I would not have done before. Even more significant, I assembled an interprofessional faculty design team at my university, beginning with cold calls to unknown faculty for a somewhat strange-sounding project. That team worked together for a year developing an interdepartmental class.

The family expert involvement in the design team was also extremely powerful for me. I renewed my commitment to persons in need and gained new, first-hand respect for their strengths and their survival skills. As a direct result of my design team participation, I sought opportunities to expand my training responsibilities by carrying my own child welfare cases in the field, which I did starting in the winter of 2000. I did this to maintain my own contact with the people we serve, to keep developing my own skills and awareness, to look for ways to make training more applicable to the field, and to reduce in some way the perceived barriers between the university and the social service agencies. One family expert with whom I worked on the design team is now serving as my "inside" source of knowledge and advice for dealing with women who are addicted to methamphetamine.

Implications for University Faculty and Courses. As mentioned above, I formed an interdepartmental, interprofessional design team among several different university departments at UNR. We spent a year meeting, learning about each other's disciplines, and developing what we determined to be the core of an interprofessional class that would help any student anticipating a career in human services. This course focused on collaborative, strengths-based, and consumer-drive service provision and was scheduled to be taught during the spring semester, 2001.

I would like to suggest several implications of such a process on a university educational system. While the faculty team participants seemed to feel very positive about the process and the experience of the team meetings, academic pressure around such issues as FTEs, tenure and promotion, and already crowded degree programs made the discussion about the specific course very complicated. I anticipate that it would be difficult to sustain true interprofessional initiatives over time in a university setting without some real commitment from key university department heads and administrators.

On the other hand, the personal relationships between faculty members begun through the design team resulted in very positive informal consultation between team members and more creative learning assignments for students. For example, one team member from a different department called me to inquire about suggestions for agency-based, community cultural experiences that I could recommend for a class she was to be teaching in cross-cultural health perspectives.

Personally, the design team experience had a profound impact on my own teaching and within my department of social work. I have made a point of including family experts as guest speakers in class. Other faculty members in my department have asked me to recommend family experts to speak in their classes. And one of the family experts and I have been invited to speak together at other classes. We speak both about her personal story as a consumer of services and as an example of how our mutual learning relationship has benefited both of us and enriched our lives. Finally, carrying cases has enabled me to relate "real life" experiences with families and social agencies that helps to make the connections between the university educational experience and professional practice much more explicit and meaningful to students.

Carenlee Barkdull's Participatory Action Research

Background. My return to graduate school in pursuit of a Ph.D. in Social Work ten years after completion of a Master's degree in the same field and a seventeen-year career in community practice was largely fueled by frustration. This frustration was both inner- and outer-directed. To provide some context, a large part of my responsibilities at my places of employment, which included local and state government and private non-profit agencies, involved collaborative work with other professionals and agencies. My roles in these collaborative human services efforts varied. At times I acted as organizer, catalyst, convener, coordinator, facilitator, funder, evaluator, or simply as participant.

Some of these efforts were more successful than others. Timing, funding, and luck certainly played important roles. My sense of inner frustration came from gaps in my knowledge, skills, and the sense that I lacked any theoretical grounding in my work. In other words, I always felt that "I was flying by the seat of my pants." And I was never sure whether I was effective or not in my various roles.

Other sources of frustration were external, and will be familiar to many readers. Chief among these was the exercise of collaboration for collaboration's sake. Frequently, the "collaboration" was created in response to pressure from funders and existed only on the grant application. Responding to concerns–often with some basis in reality–that human services operate with less than optimal efficiency in an era of burgeoning needs and inadequate resources–public and private funders adopted the new mantra of collaboration; and, collaboration became one of the most popular buzzwords of the past decade. The political and historical contexts that led to the popularity of this human services collaboration movement are worthy of treatment in a separate paper. In short, mandates to collaborate frequently were, and are, made without the understanding of local needs, contexts, and service infrastructures, and with several underlying and often misguided assumptions.

The Technical Skills I Needed and Acquired. My experiences as a doctoral student in the classroom and as a facilitator in an innovative collaborative project employing "design teams" have provided opportunities to challenge many widely-held assumptions about the nature of collaboration and various theoretical lenses through which to view my practice. As a result, I find myself with renewed faith in the value of collaborative enterprises, and have, in the process, grown as a community practitioner–and as a person.

In late 1998, I was hired as the coordinator for one of four intermountain states participating in the University of Utah's New Century Collaborative Initiative. I was able to benefit from the mentoring of a number of individuals with considerable learning and experience in the concepts and practical application of design team work. In my role, I supervised a small team of full- and part-time staff facilitating three rural sites, and personally undertook the role of faculty facilitator for a design team consisting of human services providers on one of the state's Indian reservations.

What I discovered is that I had over the years acquired and developed some skills, knowledge, and personal characteristics that proved helpful to my new role of design team facilitator. These skills included the ability to communicate verbally and in writing, problem-solving abilities, a willingness to take risks, a value for learning from mistakes and failures as well as successes, a respect for the insights of non-professionals or "lay people," and a healthy sense of humor.

What I Learned About the Design Team Process and Its Facilitation. I found myself challenged to become more sensitive to the issues of turf, but wary of my own propensity to become turf-invested. In learning to reach more effectively across professional boundaries, I had to respect the commitment to keep meetings free of jargon and learn to create safe environments where people of diverse backgrounds, experiences, and professional education could find a common language in which to frame problems and potential solutions. Explicit group norms developed and continuously modified by the design team have been enormously helpful in this regard.

While I always believed myself to be flexible and adaptable, the need to remain highly responsive to the rapidly-changing socio-political contexts and conditions in a small, rural reservation community has proved extremely challenging at times. Non-invested "critical friends" both within and outside of the community have not only provided an important means of quality control for the project, but have helped in highly personal ways as well. These friends have often helped me to regain a sense of perspective and even to re-commit myself at times when I have been personally frustrated and discouraged.

One of the most rewarding aspects of the work has been gaining some understanding of the history, cultural, social, economic, and political aspects of the community. Two colleagues have acted as cultural guides, accompanying me at many meetings to provide specific feedback, as well as acting in the capacity of cultural informants in general. A respect for the social work value of authenticity in relationships has also helped to pave the way for acceptance, as has my commitment for the 'long haul.' Design team members know that my livelihood is not dependent on their tribe's participation, nor do I receive any remuneration from the tribal government. Unfortunately, the history of Native American communities is rife with exploitation, unrealistic promises, and programs and people that disappear with shifting funding streams. The demonstration of commitment over time has been essential to the process of building trust in the community.

What I Learned About Myself and Learning. Sometimes it is difficult to tell a good day from a bad one without the benefit of hindsight. Through this journey, I have begun to understand that perhaps my primary task is to structure opportunities that help all of us internalize learning on several levels. Learning must address not only knowledge and skills, but attitudes and feelings. I believe these personally transformative experiences cannot generally take place within the standard pedagogical models under which most professionals have been schooled, nor are traditional training models typically utilized by helping agencies sufficient. At the same time, individual helpers, absent these supports, cannot successfully transform helping systems to be continuously self-examining and self-improving.

Implications: What I Learned About Collaboration. The past two years of work "in the trenches" and in the classroom have helped me to challenge many popular assumptions about collaboration, five of which I address below. Armed with new concepts and perspectives from social learning theory, organizational development theory, participatory and empowerment evaluation, and action research, I find myself equipped with new tools with which to conceptualize the work of complex community change, and my role(s) within the process.

One of the first assumptions that I had already challenged prior to returning for post-graduate studies is that people and organizations already know how to collaborate. The ability to communicate, cooperate, or even to simply co-exist is frequently confused with collaboration–working jointly with true unity of purpose. Collaboration is not simply a skill-based proposition where knowledge can be readily transferred and applied in practice. Instead, I have come to believe that collaboration is a complex set of processes and tasks that requires the creation of learning versus teaching environments. That is, we must structure settings in which participants are safe to frame and re-frame community problems, and to uncover and examine their own "theories of change"–what they believe works and what doesn't (e.g., Argyris & Schön, 1996).

The second assumption is that collaboration makes organization more efficient. This may not always be the case, particularly with the up-front investment of time and effort needed to truly develop environments of trust in which shared learning can take place and in which unity of purpose can evolve and develop. In the long run, of course, one can argue that collaboration may result in greater efficiency as professionals share expertise, agencies share resources, and consumers are required to jump through fewer hoops to receive the help they need. However, this "efficiency" assumption must be carefully examined in each context; it may not always be warranted.

The third assumption is that "experts"–professionals–know best how to re-design systems of care for better results. Design teams turn this notion on its head by bringing other kinds of experts to the table as equal partners in the change effort. Many of these experts are workers "in the trenches" and not just mid- or top-level administrators. Other experts are former or current consumers of human services, youth, elders, foster parents, or simply caring community people. The practical experience and lack of indoctrination into a profession is precisely what enables lay people to challenge the professionals at the table to think 'outside the box'–and to understand with both heart and mind how helping systems hurt as well as help.

The fourth assumption that has been challenged by my work in design teams is the notion that evaluation is some 'objective' activity that only outsiders are competent to perform. In my role as facilitator I am developing the knowledge and skills to move more fluidly between the multiple roles of facilitator, consultant, and evaluator. I am constantly trying to improve my ability to review the group's milestones in terms of process and outcomes, while simultaneously feeding this information forward as the group continues its evolving planning and implementation processes. A central role is to enlist all stakeholders in the collaboration and the community to be part of the evaluation design and process. Questions the group is now addressing include: What should we be measuring and how? What progress markers will indicate to us that we're on the right track? How do we make adjustments if we find we're not getting the results we're trying to achieve? My role, then, is one that is both empowering of stakeholders and true to many of the principles of participatory action research where success is defined and measured in ways that are meaningful and relevant to the local community (Lawson, 1999; Greenwood & Levin, 1998; Patton, 1997).

Fifth, and finally, I have had to 'unlearn' the notion that collaborative work is a linear process: one that works simply through the development of objectives, their implementation, and their evaluation. Instead I am in the process of continually re-learning that complex community change initiatives are never fixed in space and time: they are moving targets with developmental stages that may resemble a chaos textbook diagram more than a familiar flow chart.

Doing work that involves a myriad of collaborative partners and multiple, overlapping and interdependent goals has been challenging and, at times frustrating. It also has been the most rewarding work in which I have been engaged. It requires me to link community practice, research, and teaching.

DISCUSSION

When the findings from the facilitators' participatory action research are combined with the results from the interview process, several key components of the design team structure and process can be identified.

- Apparently, the design teams promoted shared thinking, the development of shared language, and the design of new collaborative practices. Shared cognition, in combination with affective and interpretive learning, yielded identical, similar, and comparable outcomes across the four states (Anderson-Butcher, Lawson, & Barkdull, in press).
- Shared thinking and outcomes were fostered by an important combination of team composition–especially the family experts– and by the skillful facilitation of faculty, including their work in creating safe, secure, and empowering activity settings.
- Faculty facilitators also learned and developed. Their participatory action research and the interview data serve to identify commonalties in their learning and development.
- Design teams need to be safe places where all participants' views and beliefs are valued and appreciated. Design team members' responses indicate that turf barriers and "professional-knows-best" attitudes cannot be left unsaid. They must be explicit learning targets in the design team process. These targets are important preconditions collaborative learning in the design teams.
- Design team members need to have ownership and be actively involved in the process.
- It is important for teams to develop a common language and mission (unity of purpose). Team process needs to focus on these important commonalties; the facilitator cannot impose them. The process of developing these commonalties is itself an important product, and it may lead to communities of practice.
- Facilitators and team members confront tensions and balancing acts. Specifically, uncertainty and ambiguity are unavoidable when new service designs and delivery systems are involved. So, facilitators and team members must effectively "normalize" some of this ambiguity and uncertainty. As one of the faculty facilitators observed, this design team work is like "building a plane while flying it" and then "flying by the seat of my pants."
- On the other hand, there appears to be a tolerance threshold or tipping point where uncertainty and ambiguity become a problem. Here, it is imperative that facilitators and team members achieve an effective balance

between exploratory learning processes and team members' perceptions of concrete tasks related to specific practice needs and problems. In other words, while the process (i.e., relationship building, turf-bashing, trust establishing, etc.) is itself an important product, teams also need tangible goals and concrete outcomes. These goals and outcomes help to engage and retain team members. They also provide a focus, helping facilitators and team members to "keep their eyes on the prize."

- Design teams and collaborative learning take time. They are not necessarily more efficient than conventional training.
- Facilitators "make or break" the design team process. They complete work behind the scenes, including retaining team members who may become impatient with the process. Facilitators must know how and when to recognize key learning and development processes and events for each team. Facilitators' also must be able to harvest key findings and lessons learned and feed them back and forward into the design team process. Without these products, team members may wonder whether they have accomplished anything of value.
- Especially in the early phases of the design team process, members are prone to see their involvement as time away from their real jobs. These perceptions indicate needs for improved linkages between changing agency expectations and job descriptions, on the one hand, and design team processes and goals, on the other.
- Faculty facilitators perform a kind of community social work related to collaborative learning and the design teams. In community settings social work practice usually includes boundary crossing, relationship building, resource mobilization, and strengths-based, solution focused interventions. These components of effective community practice are the same ones required of faculty facilitators. And, just as practice in communities depends on engaging and retaining client participation, so too, do design teams depend on the abilities of facilitators and key design team members to recruit and retain other members; and to build effective working relationships among them.
- For a host of reasons, some team members are not ready for design team participation, or for the multiple forms of collaborative practice it enables. For example, they lack the commitments, patience, and preparation for a long-term learning process surrounded by ambiguity and uncertainty, and they may not share perceptions of the need for systems and cross-systems change. Although conversion experiences occurred in some design teams, drop out was a persistent problem, and it cannot be avoided.

- The involvement of family experts was a pivotal part of the design team process, both for facilitators and for team members. Family experts have knowledge and perspectives that help professionals see themselves, each other, and their systems in new ways.
- Family experts indicated that the design team process was enriching and, in a few cases, it was described as life changing. These powerful testimonies suggest that design teams offer important contributions to the well being of family experts, including their willingness and ability to secure employment. This finding, while serendipitous, suggests that design teams may serve "clients" in ways that conventional service strategies do not.
- Because design teams are very different from conventional training, persons expecting training will voice their frustration and disappointment.
- Similarly, the initial cohort of faculty facilitators was not prepared to address the key differences between design teams as learning systems and training systems. Thanks to the evaluation and related knowledge development, future faculty facilitators can receive better preparation for their roles and responsibilities; and they also can help team members understand, from the beginning, the differences between the design team process and conventional training.
- Facilitators, like team members, also have needs for supports because design teams are new. For example, facilitators wanted and needed "critical friends" who could debrief them. Other faculty who move from training systems to learning systems also will need supports for this dramatic transition.

We conclude with a meta-evaluation finding. Design teams, systems change, and cross-systems change pose immense challenges for evaluation. For example, this evaluation utilized instruments, evaluative criteria, and methods often associated with training systems. The grants that supported this initiative required a training-oriented focus on individuals, their learning, and competency development. Although this kind of evaluation is consistent with some social learning theories, it is inconsistent with the aspects of the design team model and its learning systems.

Future evaluations should attend to team dynamics and team members' work settings. Identity and career-related dynamics and changes also require more attention.

To be sure, competency development is still important. However, competencies are merely lists. The most important evaluation criterion is the extent to which individual and group members demonstrate that powerful learning and development have occurred. Evidence in support of this learning and development is provided by measures of the extent to which they have transformed their participation, practices, identities, organizations, and institutional settings (e.g., Rogoff, 1998; Wenger, 1999). These transformations are the essence of systems change and cross-systems change.

REFERENCES

Abernathy, B. (2000, September). Introducing the work of the El Paso County, Colorado design team. Presented at the New Century Child Welfare and Family Support National Conference, Snowbird, UT.

Argyris, C. (1996). Actionable knowledge: Design causality in the service of consequential theory. *Journal of Applied Behavioral Science, 32,* 390-406.

Argyris, C., & Schön, D. (1996). *Organizational learning II: Theory, method, and practice.* Reading, MA: Addison Wesley.

Anderson-Butcher, D., Lawson, H., & Barkdull, C., (in press). An evaluation of child welfare design teams in four states. *The Journal of Health and Social Policy.*

Lawson, H. (2000, September). Training systems, learning systems, and the challenges of intervention and evaluation. National Child Welfare Conference: New Century Innovations for Vulnerable Children, Youth, and Families. Snowbird, UT.

Lawson, H.A., & Barkdull, C. (2001). Gaining the collaborative advantage and promoting systems and cross-systems change. In A. Sallee, K. Briar-Lawson, & H. A. Lawson (Eds.). *New Century Practice with Child Welfare Families* (pp. 245-270). Las Cruces, NM: Eddie Bowers.

Lawson, H., Petersen, N., & Briar-Lawson, K. (2001). From conventional training to empowering design teams for collaboration and systems change. In A. Sallee, H. Lawson, & K. Briar-Lawson (Eds.), *Innovative practices with vulnerable children and families* (pp. 361-392). Dubuque, IA: Eddie Bowers Publishers, Inc.

Rogoff, B. (1998). Cognition as collaborative process. In D. Kuhn & R. Siegler (Eds.), *Handbook of child psychology, Volume 2* (pp. 679-744). New York: John Wiley & Sons.

Wenger, E. (1999). *Communities of practice: Learning, meaning, and identity.* London & New York: Cambridge University Press.

Vital Involvement:
A Key to Grounding Child Welfare Practice in HBSE Theory

Helen Q. Kivnick
Marcie D. Jefferys
Patricia J. Heier

SUMMARY. Although children's well-being is the ultimate concern of child welfare services, the serious consequences of abuse and neglect have directed the system to a primary focus on the dangers in a child's environment. Child protective service workers have historically found little time to attend to individual and family strengths, while complying with laws and mandated procedures that prioritize minimizing harm and correcting problems. Thus, in terms of HBSE's "person and environment" duality, workers are required to attend largely to the environment and minimizing its problems, leaving them little energy for the person

Helen Q. Kivnick, PhD, is Professor of Social Work, School of Social Work, University of Minnesota, 105 Peters Hall, 1404 Gortner Avenue, St. Paul, MN 55108 (E-mail: hkivnick@tc.umn.edu).

Marcie D. Jefferys, MA, is Executive Director, Center for Advanced Studies in Child Welfare, School of Social Work, University of Minnesota, 105 Peters Hall, 1404 Gortner Avenue, St. Paul, MN 55108. (E-mail: mjeffery@che.umn.edu).

Patricia J. Heier, MSW, is affiliated with the School of Social Work, University of Minnesota, 105 Peters Hall, 1404 Gortner Avenue, St. Paul, MN 55108.

Address correspondence to: Helen Q. Kivnick, PhD, School of Social Work, University of Minnesota, 105 Peters Hall, 1404 Gortner Avenue, St. Paul, MN 55108.

[Haworth co-indexing entry note]: "Vital Involvement: A Key to Grounding Child Welfare Practice in HBSE Theory." Kivnick, Helen Q, Marcie D. Jefferys, and Patricia J. Heier. Co-published simultaneously in *Journal of Human Behavior in the Social Environment* (The Haworth Social Work Practice Press, an imprint of The Haworth Press, Inc.) Vol. 7, No. 1/2, 2003, pp. 181-205; and: *Charting the Impacts of University-Child Welfare Collaboration* (ed: Katharine Briar-Lawson, and Joan Levy Zlotnik) The Haworth Social Work Practice Press, an imprint of The Haworth Press, Inc., 2003, pp. 181-205. Single or multiple copies of this article are available for a fee from The Haworth Document Delivery Service [1-800-HAWORTH, 9:00 a.m. - 5:00 p.m. (EST). E-mail address: getinfo@haworthpressinc.com].

181

(child) and promoting her/his strengths. The child welfare field is encouraging increased attention to the well-being of children in the system. To provide a model for addressing both the person and the environment–particularly for school-aged children, this manuscript draws on HBSE theory to present vital involvement as a construct that links person and environment, and that incorporates strengths and problems. Related to popular concepts of resilience, prevention, and strength-based practice, this construct provides a basis for promoting the psychosocial strengths of children in the child welfare system, while maintaining an also essential focus on their environment. Further, the manuscript introduces practice examples that illustrate a functional distribution of professional attention between person and environment, and between negative and positive factors. *[Article copies available for a fee from The Haworth Document Delivery Service: 1-800-HAWORTH. E-mail address: <getinfo@haworthpressinc.com> Website: <http://www.HaworthPress.com> © 2003 by The Haworth Press, Inc. All rights reserved.]*

KEYWORDS. Vital involvement, resilience, prevention, strength-based practice, positive development

PERSON AND ENVIRONMENT: A MATTER OF FOCUS

Social work has historically understood human behavior as an interaction between person and environment (Richmond, 1917; Hutchison, 1999). However attending simultaneously to both elements of this interaction proves difficult for theorists and practitioners, alike. Focusing on the person, analogous to the way a cinematographer zooms in for a close-up shot of a film character, the social worker directs her/his attention to principles of individual development, psychodynamics, behavior, cognition, and the like. However, where a close-up zoom shot visually includes background material (albeit in blurred form), person-focused social work includes few integral reminders of the ongoing importance of the environment in which the person lives out her/his every moment. Indeed, person-focused social work went through a period in which it attended so fully to individual etiology and outcome that the environment all but faded from consideration.

In the reverse direction, environment-focused social work attends to elements of social systems and the physical environment, essentially ceding consideration of the unique person to scholars and practitioners in other disciplines. Calling attention to environmental influences slides, all too easily, into focusing entirely on the structure and function of multiple levels of social and physical context. The goal of this attention may, initially, be conceptualized as altering the environment *in the service of* the well-being of the person. However, in practice the ultimate well-being of the person comes, far too often, to be taken for granted, as the presumed outcome of environment-focused intervention.

HBSE, a key component of the unique scaffolding of social work theory and practice, challenges the field to maintain a dynamic balance between attention to person and attention to environment. When we bring the person into clear focus (as in theories of cognitive, moral, and emotional behavior and development), we must not lose sight of the environmental forces that continue to influence and be influenced by these personal phenomena. In evaluating person-focused interventions, we must document and consider relevant elements of the environment at the same time as we document outcomes within individual persons. Reciprocally, when we bring the environment into clear focus (as in theories of large-scale social systems (e.g., communities; social movements; political entities), small-scale social systems (e.g., families and small groups), and the physical environment) we must remember that the person endures–growing, changing, and developing in mutual interaction with that environment. Environment-level interventions impact personal processes. In evaluating environmental interventions, it is just as important (although not nearly as straightforward) to assess the resulting processes within the person, as it is to measure changes in the environment, itself.

Leading child welfare researchers, practitioners and advocates promote frameworks that attend to a child's own strengths (e.g., competencies; interests; personality characteristics), as well as the environmental assets on which the practitioner can draw (e.g., the child's family and their community). Pecora, Whittaker, Maluccio, Barth, and Bart for example, describe a model of family centered practice that used the ecological, competence-based and developmental perspectives to strengthen families so that the well-being of children can be maximized (2000). Innovative strengths-based community programs have been developed, such as the neighborhood foster care project in Portland, Oregon, established in collaboration with the Annie E. Casey Foundation. In a pilot project in Florida, a family can have its child protection case closed if someone in their community agrees to help them provide care for their children (in Waldfogel, 2000). The Casey Foundation's Family to Family Initiative, field tested in communities across the country, works to develop a network of family foster care that is neighborhood-based, culturally sensitive, and located primarily in the children's home communities (Annie E. Casey Foundation, 2002).

Nevertheless, while the benefits of focusing on children's strengths and well-being are recognized, issues of safety and permanence continue to take practical precedence, resulting in a disproportionate focus on dangers in the environment of children who are victims of abuse or neglect. Comparatively less effort is directed toward environmental supports and protections, than toward harms and risks. Less effort, still, is directed toward maximizing strengths and capacities within the child.

Part of the reason for child welfare's failure to emphasize maximizing children's strengths may be the lack of application of an appropriately comprehensive theoretical framework in practice. As McCroskey (2001) notes in her discussion of family preservation and child welfare, most of the theories on which child welfare relies ". . . focus primarily on the adult members of the family. Rather surprisingly, very little has been written about the theory base for treating maltreated children" (p 13). Resiliency theory, prevention, and strengths-based practice, all discussed later in this paper, are essential to a child welfare practice centered on child-well-being. In this manuscript, we revisit Erik H. Erikson's psychosocial theory and its construct of vital involvement (Erikson, Erikson, & Kivnick, 1986; Kivnick & Murray, 2001) as a comprehensive framework that effectively accommodates attention to person and environment, to strength and weakness. As such, we propose vital involvement as a construct that is central to HBSE curriculum and, in turn, of substantial value to a child welfare practice that attends to a balanced view of a child and her/his environment, and to the strengths and problems in each.

On the basis of HBSE theory, we argue, first, that along with targeting children's environments, child welfare practice must, at the same time, focus clearly on the psychosocial dynamics of the children it serves. We also argue that these psychodynamics include positive factors to be strengthened, as well as negative factors to be remediated. We do not disagree that child welfare practice must continue to remove children from unsafe and harmful environments, and must work to improve those environments or to replace them with more salutary ones. However, we assert that practice must focus with equal clarity on providing services that promote the development of children's psychosocial and behavioral strengths, and on documenting the increasing presence of these strengths. We provide examples of such services and clarify links between service elements, on the one hand, and elements of HBSE theory, on the other. Finally, we suggest that the outcome of child welfare practice be evaluated not only in terms of placements, reunifications, and adoptions (features of the environment), and in terms of psychosocial problems reduced or avoided (negative features of the person), but also in terms of strengths and capacities (*positive* features of the person) demonstrated in the children whose well-being is, after all, at the root of the child welfare system. This discussion is timely.

The federal government ". . . remains committed to developing child well-being measures to assess whether the child welfare system meets the health, educational and other needs of children" (U.S. Department of Health and Human Services, 2001). State governments, such as Minnesota's, are also paying increasing attention to monitoring the well-being of children in the child welfare system, along with measuring safety and permanence (Minnesota Department of Human Services, 2000). Child welfare practitioners will be best positioned to help develop and implement these indicators if they adopt practice models that explicitly incorporate goals of child well-being (e.g., strengths; growth) alongside environmental goals (parent strengths; family safety; permanent placement).

CHILD WELFARE

Child welfare in the United States is now driven by the Adoption and Safe Families Act of 1997 (ASFA) and, somewhat less directly, by the Personal Responsibility and Work Opportunity Act of 1996 (Welfare Reform). ASFA is characterized by the preeminence of child safety and health in all decision-making (McGowan and Walsh, 2000; Tracy & Pine, 2000; Kelley, n.d.). At the same time as it affirms the earlier commitment of the 1980's AACWA to family preservation and reunification, ASFA sets strict limits on these commitments. ASFA explicitly defines circumstances that pose such a serious threat to child safety that family preservation or reunification need not be attempted. In addition, ASFA mandates a permanency hearing when a child has been in care for 12 months, and it mandates the filing of a termination petition when a child has been in care for 15 of the preceding 22 months. Taken as a whole, the law essentially provides for child safety by: (1) Removing children from harmful families for up to 12 months; (2) Working with many of these families for up to 12 months to make them safer for the children to return to; and (3) Moving to safe permanent placement and/or termination of parental rights after that time. ASFA also continued funding for family preservation and support services, but gave the legislation a new name (Promoting Safe and Stable Families), reflecting emphasis on safety and permanence and requiring states to administer the programs with the safety of children as the "paramount concern" (Pecora et al., p 43).

On its face, ASFA protects children from present danger (through removal from damaging homes; through working to remediate dangerous home situations while children remain in the home), and it protects them from prolonged uncertainty and divided loyalties with regard to long-term family life (through relatively quick movement to permanent placement and termination of parental rights).[1] In dealing almost entirely with the child's environment, the child welfare system creates an artificial polarity between person and environment, rather than building on the ongoing interaction between them. The system comprises services that address a particular set of environment-based problems (those that may result in child maltreatment or delinquency). It addresses these problems by seeking to alter some features of the environment (e.g., resolve problems in troubled families; implement out-of-home placements) and to preserve others (e.g., avoid family breakup; facilitate family reunification).

Despite the growing consensus that child well-being is a core principle of child welfare services (Pecora et al.), by limiting most of its activity to determining and mitigating family-based danger, the system falls far short of achieving its proactive goal. Removing a child from an injurious setting or mitigating a setting's injuriousness reduces a measure of her/his *"ill*-being"; these changes do not, in and of themselves, promote her/his *well*-being. Further, refraining from intervening in a setting whose injuriousness does not quite reach system standards also does not promote the child's well-being. We do not question the necessity of changing the child's environment, in order to minimize damage, i.e., of intervening in the environment in order to minimize present harm and future danger to the person. Indeed, social work's grounding in the interaction between person and environment dictates that in order to promote a child's well-being, we must pay attention to more than the environment.

HUMAN BEHAVIOR AND THE SOCIAL ENVIRONMENT

HBSE in Social Work

Social work educators cite the need for a HBSE basis to social work practice (Tracy & Pine; Schneider & Netting, 1999). However we fall short as a field in adequately utilizing HBSE theory to guide the development of practice modalities, approaches, and activities that best serve the multidimensional, interacting interests of clients and their environments. This shortcoming is not unique to practitioners. Theorists seeking to understand human behavior as it develops and is expressed in the social environment tend to emphasize either the person or the environment–but not both. The same shortcoming is reflected in the system of laws and public policies constructed by policy-makers.

As suggested earlier, these person- and environment-emphases are aptly represented by the image of a movie camera. Theorists who emphasize the person (e.g., Erikson; Freud; Piaget; Gilligan; Kohlberg) bring into clear focus the specific personal dynamics or processes (e.g., psychosocial; psychosexual;

cognitive; moral) they seek to explain. To a greater or lesser extent, these theorists refer to the role of the environment in the development of the relevant set of dynamics. But even when the environment is mentioned, it remains, as in a close-up film frame, blurred and indistinct. It is present, to be sure, but as background it is all but featureless. As theorists focus on individual dynamics, so practice modalities grounded in theory comprise interventions to optimize these dynamics. (For example, psychoanalytically oriented psychotherapy seeks to directly alter pathological psychodynamics.)

Reciprocally, theorists who emphasize the environment (e.g., Bronfenbrenner; Lewin; Carter & Anderson; McGoldrick) make the environment their photographic "figure" and the person their "ground." These theorists bring into clear focus the structure and dynamics of multiple levels of the environment in which a given person lives. Or they clarify the components of social systems, and the relationships among them as part of their focus on one environmental system (e.g., family) or another. In these theories, however, individual persons and their internal dynamics remain blurred, as a film hero sitting at a desk blurs when the camera moves back to focus on the details of the photographs hanging on the wall behind him. HBSE offers social workers a vision for beginning to bring these oppositely focused bodies of theory into a productive balance, and for utilizing this balance in practice that promotes well-being in both person and environment.

Vital Involvement

The construct of vital involvement emerges from the most recent formulations of Erikson's life-cycle developmental theory which clarifies three principles to describe eight psychosocial themes as an underlying scaffolding upon which people actively–though not necessarily consciously–construct their lives (Erikson et al.; Kivnick, 1993; Kivnick & Jernstedt, 1996; Kivnick & Murray; Kivnick, in press).

According to the principle of Vital Involvement, the person enacts each psychosocial theme through characteristic behaviors and attitudes; reciprocally, life's activities, experiences, feelings, and attitudes may all be understood as part of balancing one theme or more. Psychosocial themes are meaningful only insofar as they are both psychological (related to internal feelings and capacities) and social (related to the social environment in which the psychological self exists). Vital involvement is defined as a person's meaningful engagement with the world outside the self, a process of "being in relation" (Erikson et al., p. 44) to elements of the environment (e.g., people, materials, animals, ideas, institutions, sounds) that is essential to doing internal psychosocial work and to enjoying its resulting psychosocial health (Figure 1).

FIGURE 1

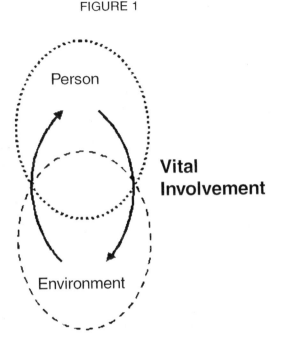

Vital involvement is the mechanism through which the person and the environment interact with and exert influence on one another. It is through vital involvement with elements of the environment that the person accomplishes the lifelong developmental work of balancing psychosocial themes. Through relationships, encounters, and activities the person essentially enacts her/his current thematic balances within terms of a unique set of environmental circumstances, and modifies those balances as the circumstances demand. The environment supports the person's development of essential psychosocial strengths in balance with their opposing tendencies–around all eight themes. An adequate or "good enough" environment supports a child's development of healthy thematic balances. An inadequate environment may fail to support the development of essential strengths while, at the same time, encouraging the emergence of excessive levels of their opposites.

For example, a home in which a baby's expressions of need are met with consistent responsiveness and care is likely to support that baby's development of a robust sense of trust balanced with mistrust. Inconsistent adult responsiveness may tilt the balance–not inappropriately–toward mistrust. The trusting, hopeful baby rewards adult attention, thereby influencing her/his interpersonal environment to remain responsive and demonstrative. Adult guidance, modeling, and encouragement support the child's development of such essential internal capacities as confidence and self-control (Autonomy & Shame/Doubt), curiosity and self-restraint (Initiative & Guilt), and perseverance in the face of initial failure or discouragement (Industry & Inferiority). Exercising these burgeoning capacities through vital involvement with specific materials, for example, prompts the child to influence her/his environment positively (by drawing lovely pictures or reading to a younger sibling) or negatively (by scrawling on a wall or hurling a book at a window). In response to positive behavior, the environment may function to encourage further mastery and experimentation.

In the other direction, a wary, mistrustful child may discourage adult attention or elicit adult antagonism. As child and parent inadvertently reinforce a cycle of negative interaction, the environment may function to strengthen the child's experiences and expressions of shame and frustration, which are likely, in turn, to continue to elicit adult responses of anger, and to develop in the child an unfortunate competence in the dynamic cycle of frustration and violence. While this child is mastering behaviors related to anger and acting out, she/he is *failing to master* behaviors related to self-control, perseverance, and problem-solving.

Vital involvement allows multiple levels of environment to influence who the person *is becoming* and how they experience themselves in the world. Reciprocally, vital involvement allows the person to express who she/he is through overt behaviors that link internal processes to entities in the external world. It characterizes any engagement (person-to-person; person-to-group; person-to-material) in which both partners have the possibility of being changed (Kivnick 2001; 2000).[2]

The construct of vital involvement encompasses HBSE's dual emphases on person and on environment. Moreover, it invokes notions of development and the lifecycle for every client. Particularly for children, we must both attend to their circumstances today and also be mindful of the connections between their experience today and their expected life involvement in the future.

Strengths and Problems

We repeat that for children involved with child welfare, we must not be concerned only with providing freedom from physical and psychosocial harm; we must also be concerned with providing environment-based opportunities for these children to develop the strengths, capacities, and competencies that will undergird their positive vital involvement– and their healthy development–for the rest of their lives. Child welfare practice has focused on developing expertise to protect children from the most serious risks and damages. However, we assert that: (1) Well-being comprises far more than a child's avoiding being either the victim or the perpetrator of dangerous behaviors; and (2) Vital involvement is a cornerstone of that "more." In addition to protecting children from harm, child welfare must be concerned with promoting the development of children's health and strengths. According to HBSE theory, such development is facilitated by providing a multiplicity of opportunities for the positive vital involvements through which a child develops psychosocial strengths, and then exercises those strengths as part of her/his community.

Influenced by the dominant medical model, two axes clarify the fields of concern primarily targeted by child welfare (Coyne, 1989), youth corrections (Clark, 1998; Brendtro & Ness, 1995), traditional youth development services (Pittman & Irby, 1996), and other forms of social work practice (Strean, 1978; Kivnick & Murray). The vertical axis identifies the location of specific concerns as ranging from the environment (e.g., physical abuse or neglect; high-violence community) to the person (e.g., depression; ADHD; violent acting out). The horizontal axis characterizes any specific concern as representing some degree of problem (e.g., present harm; fundamental need unmet; risk of harm in the future) or strength (e.g., present strength; environmental support for strength development; personal contribution to the community). The further left a concern falls on this horizontal axis, analogous to a position on a number line, the more serious the problem. The further right a concern falls, the more powerful or meaningful the strength (Figure 2).

FIGURE 2. Dominant Social Work/Child Welfare Practice Concerns

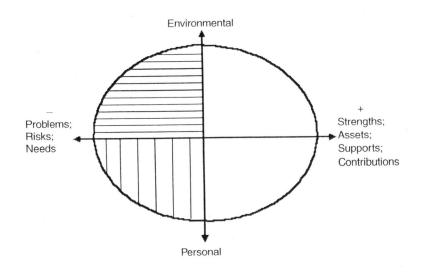

Most of child welfare practice (like conventional social work and traditional medicine) focuses primarily on concerns that fall in the left-hand quadrants. In response to concerns in the upper left quadrant, environment-based problems are identified and investigated, and interventions are implemented. The goal of this process is to diminish a problem's severity, represented by moving the position of any given concern toward the right on the horizontal axis until, at the point of the number line's origin, it ceases to be a problem altogether. For example, ongoing child abuse is reported and documented in a given family. (The family–a child's dominant microsystem–might be positioned far left on the horizontal axis.) The children are temporarily placed outside the home. Behavioral education and training are mandated for the parents. When they have progressed sufficiently that the home setting is no longer seen as unduly harmful or dangerous (the family has moved toward the number line's origin), family reunification is initiated.

Child welfare also focuses on concerns that fall in the figure's lower left quadrant. In this domain, person-based problems are addressed with the goal of lessening their severity to the point of zero. For example, a child's depression, anxiety, and acting-out behavior may be treated from a variety of psychological, social, behavioral, and pharmacological approaches. Both personal and environmental issues are addressed in order to help clients move toward a state of functioning without problems. Little effort is directed at seeking to *maximize* parent or child functioning, which would involve movement beyond the midpoint of zero, and into the right-hand quadrants that represent strengths, assets, and contributions as positive entities explicitly to be developed.

In our own personal lives, we would probably regard such *de facto* striving to achieve a state of emptiness–a state without problems or strengths–as somewhere between laughable and appalling. For ourselves and our loved ones we strive for excellence, for maximum strength, ability, and achievement. Being simply free of problems may be a starting point, but it certainly is not a goal when we consider our own lives. Why then, do we continue to practice professionally as if such emptiness were the *aim* of our work with child welfare clients?

Within the dominant medical model of clinical social work, practitioners are encouraged to regard assessed client strengths and environmental resources as mitigating identified deficits, rather than as primary bases for conceptualizing the person in her/his environment (Hepworth, Rooney, & Larsen, 1997; Strean). Indeed, dominant models fail even to provide consistent, operational language with which to discuss or measure observable client strengths or the dynamic processes that underlie them. Dominant practice models shed little light on the right-hand quadrants of Figure 2, that represent environmental and personal strengths of child welfare clients. In so doing, these models effectively constrain the system and its workers to practicing in the left-hand quadrants. We view the construct of vital involvement not only as a conceptual link between person and environment (suggested above), but also as a practical link between problems and strengths, and between practice models that focus primarily on one or the other.

Thus far we have argued both that child welfare practice focuses largely on the environment, and also that this focus seems to be largely on the environment as a source of danger and injury. In the second half of this paper, we present examples of conceptual frameworks and associated practice models that bring increased attention to the right-hand quadrants: (1) The individual child and her/his ongoing positive and negative psychosocial development; and (2) The environment (family; temporary placement; permanent placement) as an essential source of support for developmental strength and capacity incorporate some or all of these recommended domains. We conclude with visions for broader, HBSE-based practice, education, and training.

CONCEPTUAL FRAMEWORKS

Resilience

In their longitudinal study of children who survived chronic deprivations and acute traumas, Werner (1987) and Werner & Smith (1992; 1989) developed the construct of resilience to explain how some children survive in the face of horrendous risks. This construct is broadly described as the person-based ability to persevere and to achieve a good outcome, despite difficult experiences, pains, and scars. It is promoted by protective factors, described as internal and forces that help children withstand risk (Fraser & Galinsky, 1997). Resilience proponents (e.g., Masten & Coatsworth, 1998; Fraser, 1997; Garmezy, 1993; Rutter, 1990) identify personal qualities (e.g., genetic traits; developed capacities) and protective environmental features (e.g., relationships with adults; relationships *between* specific adults) that promote the resilience that enables some children to emerge, strengths intact, from extreme stresses, traumas, and deprivations. Regardless of whether determining qualities reside in the person or in the environment, resilience scholars have taught us to think of them as risk factors (that increase the likelihood of struggle and poor developmental outcomes), protective factors (that increase the likelihood of positive rebound and good developmental outcomes), and, most recently, generative factors (". . . remarkable and revelatory experiences that, taken together, dramatically increase learning, resource acquisition, and development, accentuating resilience and hardiness" (Saleebey, 1996 p. 300)).

Masten and Coatsworth point to the development of competence as a key step in the resilience model, resulting from complex interactions between the child and the adults in her/his microsystems. Their developmental discussion of resilience illustrates the principles of vital involvement, described earlier. Factors in various levels of the environment influence factors that are developing within the person. These personal factors are expressed in behaviors that both influence the ongoing evolution of environmental factors and also elicit the expression of these factors in the form of personal behaviors from significant others. Fraser and Galinsky clarify that resilience-based practice can both reduce risk and strengthen protections, and that "Intervention should mitigate risk, enhance protection, and promote resilience" p. 268.

Strength-Based Practice

In their benchmark paper, Weick, Rapp, Sullivan, and Kisthardt (1989) introduced a strengths perspective in which social workers approach clients in a spirit of collaboration, with particular concern for strengths and competencies. First, practitioners work to identify client strengths. Then they help clients develop ways to use these resources in building life solutions. Since its introduction, this perspective has come to comprise two primary elements: (1) Client empowerment; and (2) Building on client strengths (Saleebey, 1997; 1996). This perspective does not encourage the ignoring of client problems, but it ". . . demands instead that they [problems] be understood in a larger context of individual and communal resources and possibilities" (Saleebey, 1992, p. 171). The strengths perspective emphasizes client self-determination and possibility by engaging both client and practitioner in a mutual search for those personal and environmental forces that can enhance each client's life. It emphasizes the power of the person to right her/his own life course by taking appropriate advantage of resources that exist in the environment. It also allies client and practitioner around movement toward positive possibility. This powerfully motivating alliance is fundamentally different from one in which work focuses merely on moving away from problems and difficulties.

Utilizing community resources seizes opportunities for ordinary people to be vitally involved with one another, thereby promoting strength and growth in practitioners as well as in those initially identified as clients. "Emphasizing the strengths of both the person and the environment . . . can help elicit the capacities and contributions of people . . . as well as the community" (Sullivan, 1992, p. 156). Both clients and community–both persons and environment–are enriched by the development of these connections, as they stimulate one another's strengths (Benard, 1997; Saleebey, 1997). As Husock observes, this approach has much in common with the settlement house, in which people are helped through community participation, and through involvement with a broad cross-section of the population (1992). Programs are presented without being identified as solutions to problems, thus eliminating artificial distinctions between needy and helper, and enabling all interested participants to benefit.

Scholars and practitioners make use of the strengths perspective in working with such disparate populations as juvenile offenders (e.g., Corcoran, 1997; Clark; Brendtro & Ness), adult criminal offenders (Gilgun, 1999), the chronically and persistently mentally ill (e.g., Sullivan, 1997), and older adults (e.g., Stoffel et al., 2000; Fast & Chapin, 1997). Bricker-Jenkins (1997) advocates a model for public social services that is guided by a focus on strengths and resources in the client's life. Regardless of client population or specific intervention strategies, strength-based practice builds a foundation for change by: (1) Fostering (in both practitioner and client) a favorable view of the client; (2) Enabling the client first to see and then to move beyond her/his problems and diagnoses; (3) Encouraging the client to exercise existing skills and competencies; (4) Supporting the development of further client strengths; and (5) Meaningfully linking client capacities and needs to needs and supports in her/his community. As clarified on Figure 2, all five of these steps move beyond the negative, left-hand side of problem-focused practice, and they operate, quite explicitly, in terms of client strengths, environmental supports, and potential client contributions to the community.

Prevention as Positive Development

For over twenty years, the concept of primary prevention in mental health has included the complementary components of: (1) Preventing the occurrence or reoccurrence of serious disorders; and (2) Promoting healthy development (Prevention Task Panel, 1978; Cowen, 1998). The first component is consistent with Figure 2's dominant practice model in focusing on the two left-hand quadrants. By contrast, the second component focuses also on the right-hand quadrants, in keeping with the tenets of strength-based practice and the underlying values of the field of social work.

Prevention researchers identify individual-, microsystem-, and macrosystem-level factors that increase children's vulnerability to future problems, and they recommend interventions at all three levels (Resnick & Burt, 1996; Sullivan & Wilson, 1995)–targeted both at minimizing problems and also at maximizing resources. This dynamic is compatible with the construct of vital involvement as the interactive link between person and environment, driving lifelong process of positive psychosocial development. It allows us to explain what Saleebey refers to as children's "self-righting capacities" (96, p. 300) as an integral part of personal development in an environmental context.

Larson (2000) adds specificity to this discussion in describing structured, voluntary youth activities as a fertile context for positive youth development, i.e., for the development of capacities that are essential for healthy, productive functioning in contemporary adulthood. He characterizes capacity-promoting activities as (1) Intrinsically motivating to young people; (2) Stimulating young people's deep concentration or engagement; and (3) Involving a recognizable trajectory of effort toward completing a task. Notably, he points out that youth experience all three of these components far more consistently in after-school, leisure activities (e.g., hobbies; arts; organizations; sports) than in the classroom activities that constitute the school day. Motivation, concentration, and engagement are all intrinsic to the process of vital involvement. Larson's thesis points to the potential importance of after-school activities in positive youth development, and it suggests that these activities can function as crucial protections and supports in the high-risk lives of children who become involved in the child welfare system.

Conceptually related research (Jaycox, Reivich, Gillham, & Seligman, 1994) illustrates the notion of positive pathways suggested by the vital involvement construct. Children fully engage with particular activities or groups (environmental protections). In so doing, they develop a set of personal skills (personal protections) that "inoculated" them against risks, along with providing them a basis for ongoing, positive engagement.

The burgeoning field of youth work (e.g., Desetta & Wolin, 2000; Pittman & Irby) complements the conceptual frameworks of resilience and positive development, by acknowledging both that ameliorating problems is inextricably linked with promoting strengths, and also that these two processes are not proxies for one another. Particularly relevant to our construct of vital involvement is Pittman and Irby's proclamation that "Problem-free is not fully prepared" (p. 2). At the level of person, a youth who may be without serious problems is not necessarily capable either of demonstrating resilience in response to adversity, or of exercising mastery or creating success along life's ordinary path. Reciprocally, an environment that is free of major risks cannot be assumed to offer the protections and generative factors that are associated with persons' robust health and multi-faceted competence. Andrews and Ben-Arieh (1999) point to this same distinction in asserting the importance of documenting factors that promote and reflect positive development, of identifying indicators of positive human status and development, and of maintaining world-wide indices of young people's well-being.

Desetta and Wolin worked with youth in foster care, encouraging them to write about their personal strategies for self-protection and health maintenance. From these stories, the researchers identified seven resiliencies as positive person-factors among these youth at risk: Insight; Independence; Relationships; Initiative; Creativity; Humor; and Morality. These resiliencies are quite similar to the desirable youth outcomes identified by Pittman and Irby as Confidence, Character, Connection, and Competence. Whether we view these qualities as the outcomes of a long-term process of healthy youth development or as strengths developed in the midst of process, it seems clear that efforts to promote any or all of these qualities are too important to be forgotten in the midst of eliminating immediate danger, or to be left, altogether, to chance.

At the level of environment, Pittman and Irby identify seven factors as constituting key protections for youth: Stable places; Basic care and services; Healthy relationships with peers and adults; High expectations and standards; Role models, resources, and networks; High quality instruction and training; and Challenging experiences and Opportunities to participate and contribute. Bricker-Jenkins argues persuasively that the design of agency programs should reflect the assumptions of the practice model. Similarly, we assert that youth programs (e.g., education; social services; after-school activities) should be designed to provide clients these seven environment-based protections.

Vital Involvement in Practice: CitySongs

CitySongs is an after-school program in St. Paul, Minnesota, designed to promote developmental strengths through vital involvement in singing and public performance, and in relationships with consistent, competent adults. The program largely attracts children whose family situations, SES, and neighborhood factors place them at risk of child welfare involvement; it was designed explicitly to incorporate the multiple protective factors identified in the literature discussed above. The following vignette illustrates the day-to-day environment created by one particular community-based vital involvement program. It illustrates effective partnership between child protection and after-school community personnel. Sadly, it also illustrates how the failure to prioritize such collaboration can lead to the inadvertent elimination of valuable environmental supports from children in the child welfare system.

> Heaven, a serious girl of ten, and her impish brother Curtis,[3] aged eight, had just been placed in emergency foster care. The home stood across the street from the community center where the CitySongs choir practices after school. Heaven and Curtis were attracted to the lively sound of the singing, as they explored the center. Curtis immediately walked in, took a seat, and looked surprised when staff asked who he was and if he wanted to join. Heaven stood in the back and watched for quite some time before asking, quietly, if she could sit with the altos. Their foster

mother came with them to the next rehearsal and formally enrolled them in the program. She observed some rehearsals, and joined other parents in chaperoning occasional performances.

Over the next several weeks, both children found their place in the group. Curtis sang with great enthusiasm, using every muscle in his little body. He flirted with everyone. He tested every limit, and he displayed surprising docility in accepting such consequences for rule violation as having to watch a rehearsal from the sidelines, and being suspended from a performance. Heaven was far less obtrusive. She learned the alto part, and she produced both sound and silence at the appropriate cues. Although she made few overtures to the other children, she returned their smiles. And she responded eagerly when Tamika took her by the hand one day, during break, saying, "You need a friend." The two girls were inseparable after that.

After two or three months, the foster mother returned to rehearsal, to tell us that the following week the children were being moved to a long-term placement in a distant part of the metro area. She had no idea whether the new foster mother would be able to transport them to CitySongs or not. But we should know that this rehearsal might be their last with us. Heaven had just begun to work on a solo for our Spring Concert.

Their social worker told us it was too bad the kids had to leave now. CitySongs had become an important focus for their life. Heaven, in particular, was smiling and talking more. She seemed less wooden and more like a child. The social worker could not give our staff the new family's name, phone number, or address, but she promised to ask them to call us. They never did.

When I said goodbye to Heaven, I told her I was proud of how she'd made friends, how quickly she'd learned the music, and how hard she was working on her solo. She nodded. I told her we'd all miss her; she was already an important member of the group. She nodded again. But she said nothing. I broke the silence with an attempt at humor. "Are you going to say goodbye to me, or are you just going to stand there and look cute?"

Heaven looked at me with an expression of complete surprise. "Curtis is the cute one," she said. "Nobody ever says *I'm* cute!" She buried her head in my jacket. When she emerged she was serious again. "Will you really miss me? Did you really mean *I'm* cute?"

The social worker promised to mail the new foster parents a letter from our staff, asking if we couldn't figure out a way to help Heaven and Curtis remain with our program at least through this school year. Still we heard nothing. The social worker said she'd told the new foster parents about how well the children had done in CitySongs, and how much they had grown in a relatively short time. But as long as the parents complied with licensing requirements, they were free to facilitate–or not facilitate–the children's involvement in whatever community activities they chose. She could do no more than recommend that they be in touch with us. (CitySongs, 1993)

This vignette illustrates many examples of vital involvement and growth in Heaven, Curtis, and the CitySongs program, itself. Indeed, this reciprocity of positive influence–from environment to person, and back again–is precisely what vital involvement promotes, according to Figure 1. Heaven and Curtis took the initiative to engage with CitySongs in the first place. Staff welcomed them in a way that respected both their initiative, and also their right to control the pace and the degree of their involvement. In the context of their temporary group home environment, CitySongs provided a supplementary opportunity for competence, and for peer contact–one that was unrelated to family problems. The emergency foster mother supported Heaven and Curtis' initiative, in coming to enroll them in the program. She supported their ongoing participation by observing rehearsals and chaperoning performances. She supported their individual growth by cooperating with staff around Curtis's suspension, and spending time at home working with Heaven on her solo.

Heaven received regular praise from staff for the high quality of her participation. CitySongs had become a setting she could attend with regularity. Rules and expectations were clear and easy for her to meet. Her success in this system was recognized and experienced as rewarding. More important, though, were three other kinds of growth: (1) Heaven was challenged to increase her competencies around singing; (2) She developed collaborative, friendly relationships with other CitySongs Kids; and (3) She became an important member of the group. She proudly called herself a CitySongs Kid. CitySongs was stronger for her presence. In CitySongs, Heaven's identities were not those of out-of-home child, Curtis' more responsible older sister, or victim of various kinds of abuse–all roles based on problems and injuries. In CitySongs, her identities included competent singer, reliable participant, pleasant person, eager learner, sympathetic friend, and more.

We do not in any way diminish the power of the problems in Heaven's and Curtis' lives, or the need for services to change their environment and help heal their inner wounds. Neither, however, can we diminish the importance of the multi-faceted strengths they exercised in CitySongs, and the growth Heaven, in particular, accomplished. Her vital involvement in CitySongs built on personal strengths, enhanced personal assets, and enabled her, reciprocally, to enrich her environment. We must hope that the new foster parents supported comparable vital involvements in the children's new community.

It is easy to pay lip service to the adage that child welfare children are more than their circumstances. In the absence of regulations and mandated procedures to promote personal strengths in youth, however, it is both far too easy for child welfare personnel to concentrate on fulfilling mandates to solve existing problems, and far too difficult for these same personnel to implement person-focused, strength-promotion interventions. Heaven and Curtis came to–and abruptly left–CitySongs for reasons that had nothing to do with their progress or problems with the program. Had community-based protective or generative factors been eliminated when they were first removed from the family home? Were other newly-established supports being severed around this second move? How much encouragement were the new foster parents receiving, to engage environmental assets in the service of promoting Heaven's and Curtis' resilience? How well were they prepared to support meaningful vital involvement for each child? How well equipped was the child welfare system to monitor these children's vital involvement, resilience, or ongoing psychosocial health?

Having been at least temporarily removed from a dangerous home, Heaven and Curtis will make their own way through life on the basis of internalized resiliencies–developed, quite naturally, as a part of their vital involvement with activities they care about, people they like and trust, ideas they find intriguing, skills they develop, groups they choose to join and to leave, and more. For all youth, the likelihood of such vital involvement is enhanced by an environment that is–whatever its shortcomings–rich in protective and generative factors, i.e., in opportunities for vital involvement.

VISIONS FOR THE FUTURE

The vision we propose for child welfare practice is recognized by leaders in the field, partially applied in such innovative programs as Family to Family, and utilized by sensitive individual practitioners, but it has yet to be implemented as a matter of standard practice. That is, the entire area represented in Figure 3 needs to be part of social work preparation, and of practice with youth in the child welfare system. On the vertical axis, we envision practice that explicitly attends both to the child *and also* to multiple levels of the environment. On the horizontal axis, we envision practice that strives both to remediate problems and eliminate risks, *and also* to promote strengths, competencies,

FIGURE 3. Envisioned Child Welfare/Social Work Practice Concerns: Grounded in HBSE

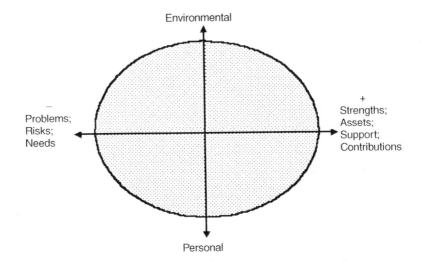

supports, and contributions. Where we earlier identified dominant practice as concentrating on concerns that lie primarily in the two left-hand quadrants, our vision for the future is of child welfare practice that attends equally to concerns that lie in all four quadrants, and to the connections among them. Interventions like those noted along with the conceptual frameworks discussed above exemplify practice in the right-hand quadrants. This major shift in practice orientation will only be effective if it is accompanied by corresponding shifts in goals articulated and outcomes evaluated. Inevitably, such a shift will lead to the emergence of new, more effective practice modalities, and an administrative system that is capable of monitoring their effects on the well-being of young people and their environments.

We envision the addition of programmatic attention to specific elements of well- and ill-being of child welfare children, and to meaningful environmental supports for children in families, in out-of-home placement settings, in families that participate in reunification, and in adoptive homes. At the same time as child welfare workers investigate possible abuse and neglect in a given home, they will also identify specific protective factors and generative factors in the child's family, school, and neighborhood environments. Problem-solving and remedial work with the family will *also* focus on maintaining and strengthening these protections–regardless of where the child resides. A major criterion for foster homes and adoptive homes will be the explicit presence and density of environmental protective and generative factors. Whether temporary or permanent, a child's placement will involve plans for maintaining or substituting specific supports from the home environment, and for introducing new supports that were absent in the home. Strengthening the child's vital involvement will be an explicit goal of placement and associated planning, rather than a serendipitous accompaniment.

When a child comes to the attention of the child welfare system, workers will assess her/his person-based strengths and weaknesses. Whatever the child's residential circumstance (environment), child welfare services will include interventions to build on the child's existing personal strengths, to remediate existing personal problems, and to work at building essential personal capacities that are not currently present. Continued involvement in out-of-school activities will be a high priority for children in the system, rather than an option that responsible adults can more easily ignore than embrace. Involvement in programming that actively builds children's personal capacities (e.g., academic; athletic; artistic; social) will be mandated and monitored, rather than recommended and then neglected. Success will be evaluated less in terms of placements finalized, and more in terms of children demonstrating increased personal strengths and capacities.

If practice is to address both person and environment, and both problems and assets, practitioners must be thoroughly trained and prepared in all four domains, as well. According to this vision, the social work methods curriculum will include strength-, resilience-, and positive development-based modalities in equal measure with the problem-focused approaches that now dominate. Students will be encouraged to consider all interventions (e.g., direct practice; policy) in terms of the strength and problem focus experienced by practitioner and by client. The history curriculum will be modified both to include social work's positively focused past, and also to reflect on the strength- and asset-focus (both explicit and implicit) of the field's major thrusts. The policy curriculum will provide students with the tools they need to analyze laws and policies for their capacity to encourage or discourage building upon the strengths of individuals, families and the community, and maximizing their expression. The research curriculum will be expanded to include existing methods for measuring and studying positive assets and resilience, and to develop new, more appropriate methods to fill current gaps. The HBSE curriculum will continue to provide a fundamental theoretical foundation for direct practice and policy. However, HBSE principles can only meaningfully inform practice if they are taught as essential to all levels of practice. This teaching must inform the presentation of HBSE content, itself, and the presentation of practice, history, policy, and research, content, as well.

Child welfare policies and regulations will be altered so that goals include demonstrating person- and environment-based strengths, along with removing problems, harms, and risks. Instruments will be adapted (and, where necessary, developed) to facilitate initial assessment and ongoing evaluation of these new factors. Practitioners will receive appropriate training and support to broaden their scope from problems in the child's environment (upper left quadrant), primarily, to include strengths the other three quadrants, with equal facility.

To comply with ASFA, workers must begin permanency planning quite early in a child welfare case. To comply with our proposed HBSE vision, they must also be sufficiently steeped in such conceptual frameworks as those presented in this paper, that permanency planning, reunification efforts, and temporary placements are all designed to promote personal strengths and capacity. In HBSE's dual focus on person and on environment, social work has a robust theoretical foundation for child welfare practice–and for all other areas of practice, as well. The construct of vital involvement helps clarify the nature of the reciprocal links between any particular person and her/his multi-layered environment. It is our task in child welfare practice to utilize these existing foundational structures to build practice systems that promote, for *all* persons, the "healthy-person-in-a-healthy-environment" paradigm that is a *sine qua non* for true social justice.

NOTES

1. One consequence of this protection is that families have a strictly limited time period in which to resolve the problems that led to placement: not all problems can be adequately resolved within this period. Another consequence is that while being protected from one set of dangers, children are likely to be subjected to a new set of risks related to the severing of emotional ties, the disruption of their social and community life, and the arbitrary imposition of new relationships.

2. The construct of vital involvement has much in common with what the field of Occupational Science refers to as "occupation," or "meaningful chunk of activity" (Clark et al., 1996; Jackson, 1996).

3. Not their real names.

REFERENCES

Andrews, A. B. & Ben-Arieh, A. (1999). Measuring and monitoring children's well-being across the world. *Social Work. 44(2)*, 105-115.

Annie E. Casey Foundation. (2002). Retrieved January 18, 2001, from <*http://www.aecf. org/familytofamily/index.html*>.

Benard, B. (1997) Fostering resilience in children and youth: Promoting protective factors in the school. In D. Saleebey (Ed.), *The strengths perspective in social work practice* (2nd ed., pp. 167-182). New York: Addison-Wesley Longman, Inc.

Brendtro, L.K., & Ness, A.E. (1995). Fixing flaws or building strengths? *Reclaiming children and youth: Journal of emotional and behavioral problems, 4*(2), 2-7.

Bricker-Jenkins, Mary (1997). Hidden Treasures: Unlocking strengths in the public social services. In D. Saleebey (ed.). *The Strengths Perspective in Social Work Practice* (2nd ed., pp 133-150). New York: Addison-Wesley Longman, Inc.

Bronfenbrennen, U. (1979). The Ecology of Human Development, Cambridge: Harvard University Press.

CitySongs (1993) [Staff participant-observation notes and reflections]. Unpublished material.

Clark, M.D. (1998). Strength-based practice: The ABC's of working with adolescents who don't want to work with you. *Federal Probation, 62*(1), 46-53

Corcoran, J. (1997). A solution-oriented approach to working with juvenile offenders. *Child and Adolescent Social Work Journal, 14*(4), 277-288.

Cowen, E.L. (1998). Changing concepts of prevention in Mental health, *Journal of Mental Health, 7*(5), 451-461.

Coyne, P. (1989). Testimony on the systematic problems of child protective services. Unpublished presentation to the Minnesota State Legislature, 11/9/89.

Desetta, A., &Wolin, S. (2000). *The struggle to be strong: True stories by teens about overcoming tough times.* Minneapolis, MN: Free Spirit Works.

Erikson, E.H., Erikson, J.M., & Kivnick, H.Q. (1986). *Vital Involvement in Old Age.* New York: W.W. Norton, Inc.

Fast, B. & Chapin, R. (1997). The strengths model with older adults: Critical Practice components. In D. Saleebey (Ed.,), *The strengths perspective in social work practice* (2nd ed., pp. 115-132). New York: Addison-Wesley Longman, Inc.

Fraser, Mark W. (1997). The ecology of childhood: A multisystems perspective. In M.W. Fraser (Ed.). *Risk and resilience in childhood: An ecological perspective* (pp 1-9). Washington, DC: NASW Press,.

Fraser, Mark W. & Galinsky, Maeda J. (1997). Toward a resilience-based model of practice. In M.W. Fraser (Ed.). *Risk and resilience in childhood: An ecological perspective* (pp 265-275). Washington, DC: NASW Press.

Garmezy, N. (1993). Children in poverty: Resilience despite risk. *Psychiatry. 56,* 127-136.

Gilgun, J.F. (1999). CASPARS: New tools for assessing client risks and strengths. *Families in Society: The Journal of Contemporary Human Services, 80,* 450-458.

Hepworth, D.H., Rooney, R.H. & Larsen, J.A. (1997). *Direct Social Work Practice: Theory and Skills* (5th ed.). Pacific Grove, CA: Brooks/Cole.

Husock, H. (1992). Bringing back the settlement house. *Public Interest, Fall 1992,* 53-72.

Hutchison, E.D. (1999). *Dimensions of Human Behavior: Person and Environment.* Thousand Oaks, CA: Pine Forge Press.

Jaycox, L.H., Reivich, K.J., Gillham, J., & Seligman, M.E.P. (1994). Prevention of depressive symptoms in school children. *Behavior Research and Therapy, 32*(8), 801-816.

Kelley, M. (n.d.). Highlights of Minnesota's New Child Welfare Law. Retrieved October 5, 1998, from <*http://ssw.che.umn.edu/cacsw/various%20Articles/highlights/pdf*>.

Kivnick, H.Q. (in press) Vital involvement: A key to personal growth in old age. In L. Kaye (ed.). *Perspectives on Productive Aging: Social Work with the New Aged.* Washington, D.C.: NASW Press.

Kivnick, H.Q. (2001). Resilience and aging. [Videotape, produced for the series Building Resilience Across the Life Cycle]. St. Paul, MN: Minnesota Department of Health.

Kivnick, H.Q. (2000, April). Old age in 2050: How aging might look from a life-span perspective. Paper delivered on Keynote Panel, Millennium Conference, Minnesota Gerontological Society, St. Paul. MN.

Kivnick, H.Q. (1993). Everyday mental health: A guide to assessing life strengths. *Generations, 17*(1), 13-20.

Kivnick, H.Q. & Jernstedt, H.L. (1996). Mama still sparkles: An elder role model in long-term care. *Marriage and Family Review, 24*(1,2), 123-164.

Kivnick. H.Q. & Murray, S.V. (2001). Life Strengths Interview Guide: Assessing elder clients' strengths. *Journal of Gerontological Social Work, 34*(4), 7-32.

Larson, R.W. (2000). Toward a psychology of positive youth development. *American Psychologist, 55*(1), 170-183.

McCroskey, Jacquelyn. (2001). What is family preservation and why does it matter? *Family preservation journal, 5*(2), 1-24.

McGowan, B.G., & Walsh, E.M. (2000). Policy challenges for child welfare in the new century. *Child Welfare, 79*(1), 11-27.

Masten, A.S., & Coatsworth, J.D. (1998). The development of competence in favorable and unfavorable environments: Lessons from research on successful children. *American Psychologist, 53*(2), 205-220.

Minnesota Department of Human Services. (n.d.). Measuring our performance and well-being of children: Indicators to help strengthen Minnesota's child welfare system. Retrieved May 15, 2000, from <*www.dhs.state.mn.us/childint/Research/ChdWelfareBk.pdf*>.

Pecora, P., Whittaker, J., Maluccio, A., Barth, R., & Bart, R. (2000). *The child welfare challenge: Policy, practice and research* (2nd edition). New York: Walter de Gruyter, Inc.

Pittman, K., & Irby, M. (1996). Preventing problems or promoting development: Competing priorities or inseparable goals? [Monograph]. *Programs that Work: What Is Youth Development.* Washington DC: International Youth Foundation. Downloaded from International Youth Foundation Web Site, 3/30/01.

Prevention Task Panel (1978). *Task panel report submitted to the President's Commission on Mental Health* (Stock No. 040-000-00393-2). Washington, DC: US Government Printing Office.

Resnick, G. & Burt, M.R. (1996). youth at risk: Definitions and implications for service delivery. *American Journal of Orthopsychiatry, 66*(2), 172-188.

Richmond, M. (1917) *Social Diagnosis.* New York: Russell Sage.

Rutter, M. (1990). Psychosocial resilience and protective mechanisms. In J. Rolf, A.S. Masten, D. Cicchetti, K.N. Nuechterlein, & S. Weintraub (Eds.), *Risk and protective factors in the development of psychopathology* (pp. 181-214). Cambridge: Cambridge University Press.

Saleebey, D. (1997 The strengths perspective: Possibilities and problems. In D. Saleebey (Ed.), *The strengths perspective in social work practice* (2nd ed., pp. 231-245). New York: Addison-Wesley Longman, Inc.

Saleebey, D. (1996). The strengths perspective in social work practice: Extensions and cautions. *Social Work, 4*(3–May), 296-305.

Saleebey, D. (1992). Possibilities of and problems with the strengths perspective. In D. Saleebey (Ed.), *The strengths perspective in social work practice* (2nd ed., pp. 169-179). New York: Addison-Wesley Longman.

Schneider, R.L. & Netting, F.E. (1999). Influencing social policy in a time of devolution: Upholding social work's great tradition. *Social Work, 44*(4) 349-357.

Stoffel, S., Kivnick, H.Q., & Hanlon, D. (2000). *Vital Involvement Groups: Piloting an Approach to Personal Strength in Old Age.* Paper presented at the meeting of the Gerontological Society of America, Washington, DC.

Strean, H.S. (1978). *Clinical Social Work: Theory and Practice.* New York: Macmillan.

Sullivan, R. & Wilson, M.F. (1995) New directions for research in prevention and treatment of delinquency: A review and proposal. *Adolescence, 30*(117) 1-17.

Sullivan, W. P. (1997). On strengths, niches, and recovery from serious mental illness. In D. Saleebey (Ed.), *The strengths perspective in social work practice* (2nd ed., pp. 183-198). New York: Addison-Wesley Longman, Inc.

Sullivan, W. P. (1992). Reconsidering the environment as a helping resource. In D. Saleebey (Ed.), *The strengths perspective in social work practice* (pp. 148-157). New York: Longman.

Tracy, E. M., & Pine, B. A. (2000). Child welfare education and training: Future trends and influences *Child Welfare, 79*(1) 93-113.

U.S. Department of Health and Human Services. (2001). *Child welfare outcomes 1998: Annual report.* Washington, D.C.: Administration on Children, Youth and Families Children's Bureau.

Waldfogel, J. (2000). Reforming child protective services. *Child Welfare, 79*(1) 43-57.

Weick, A., Rapp, R. C., Sullivan, W. P., & Kisthardt, W. (1989). A strengths perspective for social work practice. *Social Work, 34*(July), 350-354.

Werner, E. E. (1987). Vulnerability and resiliency in children at risk for delinquency: A longitudinal study from birth to young adulthood. In J. D. Burchard & S. N. Burchard (Eds.), *Prevention of delinquent behavior* (pp. 16-43). Newbury Park, CA: Sage.

Werner, E. E., & Smith, R.S. (1989). *Vulnerable but invincible: A longitudinal study of resilient children and youth.* New York: Adams, Bannister and Cox.

Current Challenges and Future Directions for Collaborative Child Welfare Educational Programs

Christina Risley-Curtiss

SUMMARY. This paper presents a brief overview of the Title IV-E and 426 investments in schools of social work that are presented in this special collection and discusses current and future challenges and issues for building effective educational programs for child welfare practice. Recommendations for future research and educational agendas are also presented. *[Article copies available for a fee from The Haworth Document Delivery Service: 1-800-HAWORTH. E-mail address: <getinfo@haworthpressinc.com> Website: <http://www.HaworthPress.com> © 2003 by The Haworth Press, Inc. All rights reserved.]*

KEYWORDS. Child welfare, retention, Title IV-E

Recruiting and retaining competent staff to serve children and families in adoptions, child protection, foster care, family preservation and support programs presents a tremendous challenge and there is a critical need for us to re-

Christina Risley-Curtiss, PhD, MSSW, is Associate Professor at Arizona State University School of Social Work, Tempe, AZ 85287-1802.

The author wishes to thank Evie Smith for her helpful comments on an earlier version of this manuscript.

[Haworth co-indexing entry note]: "Current Challenges and Future Directions for Collaborative Child Welfare Educational Programs." Risley-Curtiss, Christina. Co-published simultaneously in *Journal of Human Behavior in the Social Environment* (The Haworth Social Work Practice Press, an imprint of The Haworth Press, Inc.) Vol. 7, No. 1/2, 2003, pp. 207-226; and: *Charting the Impacts of University-Child Welfare Collaboration* (ed: Katharine Briar-Lawson, and Joan Levy Zlotnik) The Haworth Social Work Practice Press, an imprint of The Haworth Press, Inc., 2003, pp. 207-226. Single or multiple copies of this article are available for a fee from The Haworth Document Delivery Service [1-800-HAWORTH, 9:00 a.m. - 5:00 p.m. (EST). E-mail address: getinfo@haworthpressinc.com].

double our efforts towards recruiting and retaining professionally educated social workers in public child welfare (U.S. Advisory Board on Child Abuse and Neglect 1995). In addressing this need, many state child welfare agencies have turned to Title IV-E and Title IV-B Section 426 funding and schools of social work. This article presents a brief overview of those efforts, to date, including those highlighted in these two special issues, and of current and future issues facing agency-school partnerships; and suggests recommendations for future research and educational agendas.

STAFFING CHILD WELFARE AGENCIES

Current educational and training needs for child welfare practice have their roots in the growth of demand for services that has taken place both nationally and at state levels; and in the increasingly complex situations that families entering the child welfare system bring with them. The demand is reflected in the enormous rise in numbers of reports of child maltreatment received by child welfare agencies, and of subsequent out-of-home placements. For example, between 1980 and 1995 the number of children reported to be abused and/or neglected increased 258.3%: from 1.2 million to 3.1 million (Petit & Curtis, 1997; National Center on Child Abuse and Neglect, 1997). The number of children living in out-of-home care increased from approximately 302,000 in 1980 to approximately 483,000 in 1995; a 59.9% increase (Petit & Curtis, 1997, American Public Welfare Association, 1997).

The increasing complexity of child welfare client situations is seen in the numbers of families with multiple complicated problems. These include, for example, the co-occurrence of substance abuse and child maltreatment. An estimated 60-81% of families reported for child maltreatment have alcohol or drug problems (Young, 2000; Prevent Child Abuse America, 1996). Addiction to alcohol and other drugs can be a chronic, relapsing disorder with recovery a very long term process. While addiction is the most common co-occurring problem, it is rarely the only serious problem: poverty, substandard housing, mental illness, domestic violence, animal abuse and HIV/AIDS are also often present (Lawson, Anderson-Batcher, Petersen, & Barkdull, 2002; U.S. Department of Health and Human Services, 1999). Since 1970 the percentage of children living with both natural parents has decreased and the poverty rate for families with children has increased. In addition, research in recent decades has increased our knowledge regarding our understanding of the complex interaction of factors that occur in maltreating families.

Nationally, the increase in demand and complexity has been felt throughout the child welfare system, resulting in acute shortages of professionally trained staff in public child welfare agencies. According to a General Accounting Office (1995) report, in response to an APWA survey, 90% of states reported difficulty recruiting and retaining caseworkers. In 1996, Taunton County, Massachusetts reported a 100% turnover and in 1997 Broward County, Florida reported an 85% turnover rate (Jordan Institute for Families, 1999). This makes staffing the most serious issue, next to funding, facing these child welfare systems (General Accounting Office, 1995).

More specifically, in Arizona, a wide gap developed between the demand for child welfare services and the availability of qualified staff to meet this demand. Because of personnel shortages, the Department of Economic Security (DES) was, in some recent years, unable to respond to as many as 25% of child abuse and neglect reports deemed appropriate for investigation statewide. In the state's two most populous counties, the rate of uninvestigated reports at one point exceeded 33% (Arizona Supreme Court Foster Care Review Board, 1987). Though new funds were made available to add positions, the lack of qualified applicants has often thwarted efforts to improve services. Unfortunately, in many states a partial solution has been to restructure and redefine the intake and investigation process so as to reduce the number of reports that are counted as reports. In Arizona, for example, reports screened as lower risk are not investigated but rather are referred to Family Builders as part of a strategy to investigate 100% of the reports to the centralized hotline. In addition, difficulty in recruiting trained staff has contributed to the deprofessionalization of public child welfare positions (see e.g., O'Neill, 2001).

Historically, the issues of child welfare have been a major focus of social workers. For example, a settlement house for children was established in 1887 in New York City (Levine & Sallee, 1999). The 1920's embrace, by social workers, of the casework method and individual treatment was reflected in child welfare agencies where these became the major intervention components (Mather & Lager, 1999). In fact, professionalization of a public child welfare work force was viewed as desirable and many states and counties, in the 1920s and 1930s sought out child welfare workers with social work education and experience (Leighninger & Ellett, 1998). Also in the 1920s, social worker Grace Abbott headed up the Children's Bureau in Washington, DC and her sister, Edith, conducted research on juvenile delinquency, child labor, housing conditions of the poor and employment of women (Popple & Leighninger, 1999). Edith Abbott and Sophonisba Breckinridge helped establish the School of Social Service Administration at the University of Chicago–a social work program with primarily a focus on public welfare.

In the 1930s, federal funding was made available for social work education of public child welfare workers through the Social Security Act. The Children's Bureau was put in charge of child welfare grants to states and encouraged to work with public child welfare agencies to strengthen services especially in rural areas. The Bureau encouraged professionalism of employees and made child welfare grant money available to agencies for granting educational leave to workers for attendance at recognized schools of social work. As of 1939, at least 35 states and Hawaii had granted educational leave to people to attend graduate schools of social work (Leighninger & Ellett, 1998).

In fact, schools of social work and child state child welfare agencies have been collaborating for some 60 years (Zlotnik, 1997). However while the social work profession has had a great influence on child welfare and has been the dominant profession in child welfare, this connection has 'waxed and waned' (Zlotnik, 2002). In the last two decades, in particular, it appears that the social work profession has, to a large extent, forsaken child welfare (Kravitz, 1992). While in the 1950s approximately 50% of staff were professional social workers (Leighninger & Ellett, 1998), almost half the states responding to a 1987 national survey did not require entry-level child welfare workers to have completed even baccalaureate degrees in order to hold direct service positions (Russell, 1988). In addition, while 37% of states responding to the study did require a college degree, none mandated that entry-level workers have a social work degree. Another study of 5,000 child welfare staff showed that only 28% had BSW or MSW degrees (Lieberman, Hornby, & Russell, 1988). Much more recently, a member survey by the National Association of Social Workers (NASW) found that only 8% had child welfare/family as their primary practice area and only 6% identified government agencies as their primary employer (NASW, 2001a).

Arizona was one of the states in which the elimination of degree requirements for child welfare positions occurred, and statistics on Arizona Department of Economic Security (DES) staff provide evidence of deficiencies in worker education across the state. In 1994, over 12% of DES child welfare workers did not have a college degree (National Resource Center for Child Welfare Management and Administration, 1994). Those who did have college educations were most likely to have undergraduate degrees in fields other than social work (34%). Only 15% held an MSW degree, and 9% had a BSW degree. In too many states this situation continues.

AGENCY-UNIVERSITY PARTNERSHIPS

A number of federal policies, as highlighted in several articles in this special volume, have helped to rejuvenate efforts to professionalize (i.e., reprofessionalize) public child welfare by making specific funds available for agency partnerships with schools of social work for professional development of child welfare workers. Chief among these policies, outlined by Zlotnik in her articles "The Use of Title IV-E Funds for Social Work Education: An Historical Perspective, " and " Preparing Social Workers for Child Welfare Practice: Lessons from an Historical Review of the Literature" are the 1962 Amendments to the Social Security Act and the Child Welfare and Adoption Assistance Act of 1980 (P.L. 96-272). The 1962 Amendments to the Social Security Act created Title IV-B Section 426. This is a discretionary grant program which provides monies for undergraduate and graduate education, support of short-term in-service training for current public child welfare agency employees, and curriculum development. In 1997, the Children's Bureau awarded 3 year grants to 23 social work education programs, in 1998 with a $2 million increase it awarded 29 new grants. 1999 again saw an increase in Section 426 funding, up an additional $1 million for a total of $7 million (Council on Social Work Education, 1999). Examples of Section 426 grant priorities have included : interdisciplinary training for public agency workers and supervisors to improve child welfare services; training child welfare managers to support outcome-based management (Council on Social Work Education, 1998); professional education for awarding BSW and MSW degrees to prospective entry level, and existing, public child welfare agency staff; professional education for prospective and current American Indian and/or Alaska Native students enrolled in BSW or MSW programs; and training for frontline child welfare staff to prevent child abuse and neglect (Council on Social Work Education, 1999). (See in this volume Grossman & McCormick, and Lawson et al.)

Especially helpful to reprofessionalization efforts has been the Title IV-E program created by P.L. 96-272. This program provides funding for states to train current public child welfare staff or those preparing to become employees of those agencies. Unfortunately while P.L. 96-272 was passed under President Carter the implementation and funding fell to the conservative Reagan administration. With an emphasis on limiting government involvement and funding in social services many of the Act's provisions and regulations were not instituted (Leighninger & Ellett, 1998; Zlotnik, 2002). For example, regulations for P.L. 96-272 which supported BSW degrees for line workers and MSWs for supervisors as minimum qualifications were never released (Leighninger & Ellett, 1998). In addition, the Children's Bureau staff was drastically cut and they were unable to keep abreast of the new developments such as provision of Title IV training funds (Zlotnik, 2002).

The 1990s brought a new administration and a less conservative federal philosophy. Staff at the Children's Bureau became aware of Title IV-E's potential and began encouraging its use. Despite its slow start and inconsistent interpretations of Title IV-E regulations, this program has been accessed to fund a variety of additional efforts on the part of public child welfare agencies and schools of social work to improve child welfare services. These efforts include: a Public Child Welfare Certification Program for recruitment of BSW students provided through a consortium of universities in Kentucky (Fox, Miller & Barbee, 2002); support for current child welfare employees to get their MSWs in Texas (Scannapieco, Connell and Granger, 2002) and Minnesota (Wattenberg, 1998); support for BSW or MSW education to prepare potential child welfare workers in Louisiana (Gansle & Ellett, 1998); child welfare curriculum development efforts in California (Coleman & Clark 2002; Clark, 2002) and educational support for MSW students in California (e.g., Jones & Okamura, 2000), Arizona (Risley-Curtiss, McMurtry, Loren, Gustavsson, Smith, & Faddis, 1997) and Washington (Phillips, Gregory & Nelson, 2002). In 1999, at least 48 schools of social work throughout the U.S. received Title IV-E funds for BSW students (Pierce, 2002) and Zlotnik and Cornelius (2000) report at least 33 MSW programs receive such funds.

CURRENT CHALLENGES
FOR PUBLIC CHILD WELFARE AGENCIES

Funding and staffing are the two most serious issues facing public child welfare agencies today. Staffing involves not just recruiting and retaining bodies but employees who are qualified to meet the challenges presented by today's children and their families. There appears to be consensus that professionally educated social workers can fit this bill. Reprofessionalizing public child welfare has significant support; both from expert opinion (see e.g., National Association of Public Child Welfare Administrators, 1987; Leighninger and Ellett,1998; Mather & Lager, 2000; Scannapieco, Connell, & Granger, 2002) and research (see e.g., Booz-Allen, 1987; Jones & Okamura, 2000; Lieberman, et al., 1988; Pecora, Briar & Zlotnik, 1989). Thus there is a need to attract individuals with BSW and/or MSW-level training into the field.

Public child welfare agencies, however, are faced with the issue that current BSW/MSWs have little incentive to consider public child welfare as a career option. Agency barriers to their recruitment and retention are well known and include: low salaries comparable to work in retail stores, movie theaters and supermarkets; lack of career ladders; inadequate supervision; and stressful work environment including an often negative bureaucratic organizational climate and excessive workloads (Alwon & Reitz, 2000; Briar-Lawson, 2001; Fox, Miller, & Barbee, 2002). In addition, there is the cost of the "emotion labor" that is necessary for case workers to make when dealing day in and day out with trauma–both vicarious and direct (Clark, 2002; Horejsi, Gaithwait, & Rolando, 1994; Horwitz, 1998).

Another challenge that child welfare agencies are currently facing is a growing diversity among the clients they serve (Clark, 2002). While non-whites, especially African-Americans, have long been over-represented in the public child welfare population they have not constituted the majority. This is changing, however, with the increased diversification of the United States and the growth in, especially, the Hispanic population. Agencies are being challenged to provide culturally appropriate services with a staff that has not followed the increasingly diverse trend.

Policy initiatives such as the Adoptions and Safe Families Act of 1997 (ASFA), the 1994 Multiethnic Placement Act and its 1996 amendment, and Temporary Assistance to Needy Families (TANF) also have created challenges for public child welfare agencies to create new service designs and delivery systems (Jordan Institute, 2000; Lawson et al., 2002). For example, when TANF replaced the Aid to Families with Dependent Children Program the social safety net for many families was gone. Short term and long term benefit limits and employment requirements created the need for assessing job-related needs and supports such as transportation and child care, and for employment interventions (Briar-Lawson, 1998). AFSA, and its newer amendments, has presented child welfare agencies with new standards for front line practice (e.g., time lines, concurrent planning, family group decision-making) and requirements for agency accountability such as outcome measures. Allocation of funding is based on compliance with reporting requirements. Each policy, alone, creates complications for child welfare agencies; in combination, given an already inundated system, their impact has been acute (Lawson et al., 2002).

Public child welfare agencies also are struggling with the issue of privatization, including pressure from state legislators to privatize. For example, in 1996 Kansas the state child welfare agency moved from providing direct family preservation, adoption and foster care services themselves, to contracting with private providers under a managed care system of capitation. The agency retained their CPS investigative functions but otherwise became a contractor and monitor of services rather than a provider (Friesen, 1999). Such a change in job focus raises multiple staffing issues including necessary qualifications needed, ethical dilemmas, and attractiveness of such jobs for professional social workers.

CURRENT CHALLENGES FOR SOCIAL WORK EDUCATION

Social work education is currently experiencing many challenges that can affect its ability to establish and maintain productive partnerships with child welfare agencies. Chief among these challenges are declining enrollment numbers, university-wide funding issues and trends such as reorganization with free standing schools being placed under combined departments (e.g., UCLA, ASU), and development of a career model of education rather than one that emphasizes a broad knowledge base and critical thinking.

For example, rapid growth in the number of social work programs (some 464 accredited or in candidacy BSW programs, 117 + MSW programs and 71 + PhD programs (Gade Web Page/ 1998; Kadushin, 1999; Piece, 2002) sharing the same declining pool of applicants is resulting in schools of social work focusing more on marketing strategies to recruit students than on providing quality professional education for service to clients. We perceive that our survival is at stake and that we exist in a student-driven marketplace. So while the world of information regarding human beings and their interactions with their environment is exploding (e.g., multi-cultural information, neural brain development, infant mental health, resilience, wellness and spirituality), and client issues are becoming increasingly complex (e.g., co-occurrence of violence, substance abuse and mental illness; dual dependency with delinquency adjudication), schools of social work are looking for ways to increase enrollment by reducing the time it takes to get an MSW degree (i.e., fewer courses in advanced standing programs), making social work education available through mechanical technology (computers, video conferencing and tapes), developing combined MSW/PhD programs, and eliminating requirements that faculty must have a minimum of two years post-MSW practice experience to teach social work practice. Faculty who teach policy and research have no such requirement.

"The socialization of students for professional practice is falling from the top to the bottom of graduate school priorities" (Cloward, 1998, p. 585) with distance education, accelerated programs, and such. "Advanced standing programs are good for recruitment but they are a marketing tool not an educational tool" (Vinton, 1999). "Graduate schools of social work, especially the better-known ones, are taking on the attributes of research institutes, with faculty venturing into the field of practice only to collect data" (Cloward, 1998, p. 584).

Another challenge for social work education is that student applicants have also changed with more students preferring to go into some form of private practice, whether it be private agency practice or self-employment (see Abramczyk, Raymond & Barbell, 1992; Costin, Karger, & Stoesz, 1996;

Hansen, 1992; Helfgott, K. 1991). With growing concerns about professional prestige the preferred client population is 'the worried well' (Leighninger & Ellett, 1998) and the preferred work environment is *not* a major child welfare bureaucracy with excessive red tape, high caseloads and frequent public harassment (Hansen, 1992). With schools of social work existing, more and more, in a student-driven marketplace they must respond to these 'needs' in order to attract students. This situation has had ramifications for schools of social work at the doctoral and new faculty levels, where there have been fewer students with child welfare backgrounds and interests, and hence a lack of new PhD faculty with those qualifications (Kravitz, 1992).

The growth of managed care, especially in the public sector, has also contributed to a turning away from public service practice where social workers are expected to be more concerned with cost containment than adequate treatment for clients, and ethical dilemmas are an every day occurrence. Managed care also presents a dilemma for schools of social work. Do we swallow our professional ethical standards and change our curriculum to accommodate cost containment as the primary goal or do we educate students to advocate against the reality of managed care and help create service delivery systems that serve clients justly. Do we lead our profession or do we follow?

The increasing ethnic diversity of our population and hence of the types of clients who need assistance also is an issue for schools. It is not enough just to 'produce' culturally competent Anglo social workers; many schools are struggling with how to recruit and retain more students of varying ethnic backgrounds.

All of the above issues raise curriculum issues for schools of social work. For example, advanced standing programs call for an abbreviated course load based upon the assumption that entering students have a certain level of knowledge and skill. In addition, much of the current BSW and MSW curriculum is 'old' in that it reflects traditional western European models of direct and indirect practice: this does not represent our increasingly diverse and complicated population. In fact, we need to be producing bilingual as well as multiculturally competent social workers. Schools are challenged then to graduate students who are well grounded in assessment and treatment (including prevention) of substance abuse and violence; skilled at critical thinking (Scannapico et al., 2002), at working with the seriously mentally ill, with interdisciplinary staff (Grossman & McCormick, 2002), and with clients from culturally diverse backgrounds; and at the provision of concrete and material goods. Unfortunately while the practice of child welfare is becoming increasingly complicated and major changes have occurred in child welfare agencies, there have been fewer changes in schools of social work.

Another curriculum issue that Schools with BSW programs have been struggling with has to do with the Council on Social Work Education's (CSWE) accreditation requirement that BSW curriculum focus on a generalist model of practice while MSW programs have an advanced specialization focus. If the minimum requirement for child welfare employment is to be the BSW degree, how can schools adequately prepare these students for specialized child welfare work?

Schools of social work are also being challenged by university pressures for more grant funded research, publication, and teaching while continuing to be a major provider of service to the community. For example, in the past few years a major university-wide focus at Arizona State University has been faculty workload with goals of increasing the number of senior faculty teaching undergraduate courses, while at the same time increasing federally funded research in order to maintain their Research I status. In addition, they have also staved off legislative attempts to determine teaching loads and program content.

Finally, schools of social work face another challenge in that unlike business schools for example, the mission of social work education is not necessarily the real mission of students. And neither the mission of the schools or of students is consistent with the public agency mission. Thus schools struggle to satisfy many constituents with very different agendas.

FUTURE DIRECTIONS
FOR AGENCY-UNIVERSITY PARTNERSHIPS

We are entering another period of conservative government–fiscally as well as socially. As it did in the 1980s (Leighninger & Ellett, 1998; Zlotnik, 2002), this can mean the reduction or end of federal initiatives for many programs including professional development in child welfare. Additionally, the extension of funding to faith-based services means more competition for limited monies, and endorsement of a service delivery system that often is staffed more by well intentioned volunteers rather than well trained professional social workers.

Given this conservative political and fiscal climate, it is even more critical that schools of social work and child welfare agencies work together to address the needs of vulnerable children. Regardless of what happens to Title IV-E funding, the programs and projects described in these pages confirm that much can be accomplished by close collaboration between federal and state agencies and among different organizations within states. There is a need, however, to institutionalize the structures and relationships established thus far in order to ensure that future changes are planful, worthwhile, and able to transcend political uncertainties.

Institutionalization

Action also is needed to institutionalize the connection between child welfare and social work. For example, the Arizona chapter of the National Association of Social Workers, ASU Schools of Social Work (Main and West campus programs) and several community advocates are exploring ways to create an ongoing coalition to advocate for the hiring of professional social workers in public child welfare as well as other public social services. Also on the local and state levels, we need a formalized process in which representatives from schools and child welfare agencies can meet regularly to exchange information, provide updates on successes and provide technology transfer.

On the national level, there is a potential network of over 75 schools/departments of social work in partnership with public child welfare agencies (Leighninger & Ellett, 1998). While grant funding has been used for IV-E Partnership newsletters and conferences we must find a way to organize a more long term, inclusive and comprehensive mechanism for communication between agencies, social work education, the social work profession, and social work practitioners themselves. Such an organization should take a leadership role in setting a national agenda including the reprofessionalization of public child welfare, the maximization of federal funding, accreditation of training curricula, issues of the gendered nature of the workforce and need for culturally congruent agency practices and policies, testing and dissemination of new management and service delivery models such as front line units as design teams, the use of family experts, multi-track CPS systems, neighborhood teams, and family to family models, and enhancing the ability of schools to prepare students for public child welfare work by creating and revising child welfare related curriculum and encouraging additional partnerships between social work education and public child welfare. The Child Welfare League of America has taken steps in this direction with their 1999 and 2001 work force conferences and the creation of a National Advisory Committee on the Workforce Crisis. Nonetheless the existence of a regular forum, inclusive of state agencies and social work educators and practitioners, for discussing, exchanging and disseminating information and ideas, and taking leadership, is needed if professionalization of child welfare is to succeed.

Mission

For such a collaboration to take place however, schools and public agencies face the challenge of creating a unifying mission (Alwon & Reitz, 2000; Chavkin & Brown, 2002) that promotes the development of a well educated and trained professional work force. Currently a primary mission of many public child welfare agencies is looking for documentable formulations so they can be absolved in the legal litigation that is becoming so common and costly; for schools of social work a primary mission is too often focused on meeting students demands in order to get more bodies (Chase & Cahn, 1992; Kravitz, 1992). Neither of these missions advances the professionalization of child welfare or quality practice with clients.

To successfully meet the challenge of creating a common mission agencies and schools will need the wholehearted support of the social work profession as embodied by such organizations as CSWE and NASW. This support has not been forthcoming given the lack of attention from, for example, NASW whose membership reflects more private agency work with the typical client being a white female 35 or older (NASW, 2001b). As for CSWE, they play at supporting the profession's involvement in child welfare: however, their commitment appears minimal when they reduce the number of Title IV-E presentations at the annual APM, and support the idea of eliminating the requirement for social work degrees for positions such as field instructors or for experience in the field prior to teaching.

Social Work

For their part, schools of social work need to reexamine and strengthen their own commitments to reprofessionalizing child welfare. Promoting social workers in public child welfare means schools must take a proactive role within their immediate and broader environments. For instance, a comment was made at the 2000 Partnership Conference in DC that social work faculty do not like public child welfare and discourage students from pursuing it for employment. While the majority of faculty may not do this, my own experience supports the idea that this does occur. Research suggests that retention of social workers in child welfare depends to some degree on commitment to the importance of child welfare work to children, families and communities (e.g., Ellett & Millar, 2001; Scannapieco et al., 2002). Thus schools need to create an educational environment that values public child welfare agency work, at least as much as any other practice area, and puts more emphasis on our social work values and Code of Ethics, both of which promote a strong commitment to working with the oppressed and underserved (i.e, much of the child welfare population).

Schools of social work need to take a hard look at their curriculums, updating and adjusting them in order to meet the changing needs of child welfare agency practice. In Arizona, DES staff identified the following knowledge and skill areas as needed in graduating MSWs seeking employment in CPS: (1) assessment and intervention especially in relation to families with issues of substance abuse, violence, and mental illness; and in relation to communities; (2) skill in writing goals, objectives, and plans; (3) knowledge of crisis management and counseling, and (4) case management; (5) computer literacy; and (6) multicultural competence. These skills and knowledges need to be encompassed in a "family-centered strengths based approach." Again, retention research suggests that workers who perceive themselves to be competent and able to successfully accomplish outcomes in child welfare are more likely to stay (e.g., Ellett, 2001; Jones & Okamura, 2000). What do schools of social work need to do to help their potential child welfare students to feel more competent than they currently do?

This DES staff input reflects concrete areas where knowledge and skills are needed. However the schools are also faced with the challenge of broadening their ways of thinking and knowing. For example, educating students to be critical thinkers and to go "outside the box" calls for an expanded paradigm that embraces many epistemologies beyond the dominant one of positivism and post positivism. Current initiatives such as family group conferencing, family experts and design teams all reflect the belief in family-centered collaboration and empowerment of clients. Unfortunately, a major obstacle in implementing family group conferencing has been the case workers' reluctance to believe that families can make good decisions, and to let go of some of their control (Lupton & Nixon, 1999). Again, schools of social work can be a force here by opening students to the infinite possibilities of our clients.

Moreover, the increasingly multicultural nature of our child welfare clientele also requires the inclusion in schools of material and experiences that defies the traditional western model of intervention (both macro and micro). Overlaying cultural information on the current western based curriculum is not enough. There is now a need to develop alternative curriculums that meet the needs of specific ethnic populations. In Arizona, for example, with its large and growing Hispanic population, there is clearly a need to develop an alternative curriculum that focuses on working with children and families who may be recent immigrants or illegal aliens, who speak little to no English, or may be related to inhabitants established here long before Arizona became a state. We also need a curriculum that focuses on working with First Nations persons. Many faculty and agency staff who engage in developing such curriculums will need to learn as they go and to be prepared to re-examine their own ideas regarding the way social work education should be taught and social work practice carried out.

Students entering the field of child welfare also must, more than ever, be prepared for interdisciplinary practice (Grossman & McCormick, 2002). This includes being able to work with staff employed in physical or mental health care, child care, law, and corrections. This collaboration comes in many forms from communication across systems, to diffusion of knowledge and service mergers. Thus curriculums and field practica must be expanded to reflect learning of relevant skills and knowledge.

Schools also need to review their field instruction models with the goal of assessing whether students are getting the best preparation they can for child welfare work. Public child welfare services field placement experience is considered vital for students planning careers in child welfare, yet many state agencies are unable to provide enough internship opportunities. This is due largely to the already high demands placed on CPS supervisors and case workers who might serve as field instructors for student interns, and to the fact that, in many states, few CPS supervisors meet criteria for being field instructors, such as holding an MSW degree. The creation of specific field units can considerably increase the number of field placements available. In addition, given that field practica are one of the best conduits for jobs in child welfare (Gomez & Harris, 1992) another benefit may be the recruitment of students into the field. A direct benefit to the agency of these units is the services it provides to clients (Risley-Curtiss et al., 1997). Given the smaller caseloads that students carry, field unit staff and students interns are able to provide more intensive and specialized services to the families in their caseloads. This also means that such field units provide a sort of laboratory or incubator for innovative practice models and service improvements. Thus the units provide an opportunity to influence practice both in the agency itself, and in the social work curriculum.

Schools of social work and agencies also need to get serious about preparing students and staff to be supervisors and in supporting them once they are supervisors. Research shows that good supervision is very important in retaining child welfare staff (Briar-Lawson, 2001; Jordan Institute for Families, 1999; Scannapieco et al., 2002); thus supervisors need to be valued by agencies for more than compliance with time lines and meeting statutory requirements (i.e, administrative managers). They need to be valued for, and able to provide competent support, education, and case work leadership. Examples of possible initiatives could include collaborative efforts to develop and implement post-MSW child welfare supervision certification programs (using IV-E and/or 426 funds?) and the inclusion of courses on public agency supervision in MSW programs. This latter recommendation, of course, assumes the expansion rather than the reduction of curriculum course requirements.

Public Child Welfare

On the agency side, research supports the need for change in the public child welfare agency organizational culture (e.g., Drake & Yadama, 1996; Ellett & Millar, 2001). Fox, Miller, and Barbee (2002) report that studies in the corporate sector have found that key aspects in recruiting and retaining talented workers are careful selection, human services management practices and a strong commitment to providing training and professional development. These companies, which were engaged in a labor war due to low rates of unemployment, have focused on creating a positive, employee-centered culture to attract and keep employees. Public child welfare agencies must follow suit if they expect to have any impact on their retention situation, and they must do more than just "talk the talk," something they have become very adept at. Schools of social work must actively support agency efforts by initiating offers to serve on planning committees and act as consultants. The ground work is already being laid as a result of the December, 1999 "Confronting the Workforce Crisis" national symposium hosted by the Child Welfare League of America. This included representatives from both agencies and social work education. From that meeting, a National Advisory Committee on the Workforce Crisis in Child Welfare was formed.

Alwon and Reitz (2000) report on the work of the recruitment and retention subcommittees which have identified themes that seem to be characteristic of organizations that successfully recruit and retain skilled, motivated staff. The themes emphasize an agency climate that "walks the walk" by having a mission that is directly linked to employee's work, with policies and decisions conforming to that mission, by strongly emphasizing open communication, relationships, partnerships, teamwork, learning, innovation and development among, and at all, levels of the organization, and by freeing employees to make decisions and take action with fewer levels of policy, procedures and bureaucracy (Alwon & Reitz, 2000). Another conference was held in May, 2001 in Texas.

In addition, several authors in these pages have pointed out the influence that the social work profession has had on public child welfare. There is a need now for public child welfare agencies to be aware of issues being discussed and addressed in the social work education arena; and to invite themselves to be part of the discourse and perhaps, part of future initiatives. For instance, agency personnel at the 2000 Partnership Conference in Washington, DC clearly voiced the desire to have input from Schools of Social Work faculty in many capacities including research, evaluation, and as committee members. Nonetheless they repeatedly emphasized that such input needed to be grounded in a firm understanding of the contextual realities of their practice (i.e., they must have had practice experience). Thus the outcome of the current debate in social work education regarding the need for practice experience for future faculty has direct relevance to the future of such input. Child welfare agencies need to be voicing these concerns to social work educators.

Research

The close of the 2000/2001 academic year marked the end of roughly a decade of Title IV-E partnerships. This means that sufficient time has passed and a sufficient number of students have graduated from some Title IV-E programs to allow for meaningful outcome evaluation. Some of these have begun (e.g., Jones & Okamura, 2000; Risley-Curtiss et al., 1997; Scannapieco et al., 2002). We need more (Chavkin & Brown, 2002), especially if we are going to successfully professionalize public child welfare with BSW/MSWs, because we need more evidence than we already have to support our contention that this is the best way to go. A more extensive research effort will be needed to address questions such as: How well are students prepared for contemporary child welfare practice and how effective are they in delivering services to vulnerable populations? What elements in the preparation and support of trained child welfare workers help to establish and maintain positive working relationships with clients and other service providers? Do stipend recipients differ from non-recipients in terms of job performance and retention, and if so, how?

Title IV-E projects provide rich opportunities for research and evaluation at the client level as well. The laboratory for this work is the field education unit, where a number of research problems can be addressed. For example, the goal of the field units in Arizona (Risley-Curtiss et al., 1997) is to allow students to provide services that come as close as possible to standards for ideal practice. This includes regular and systematic measurement, intensive contact with families, more frequent case staffings, and maximal use of collateral services. Each aspect of this ideal model can be examined and tested in the units' "laboratory" setting, and research efforts of this sort are beginning. A further benefit is that this research will itself help train students to incorporate evaluative techniques into their practice and to view service delivery and research as integrated elements rather than distinct endeavors.

There is need for research partnerships that go beyond IV-E programs. For example, we need to explore whether, in child welfare agencies, social workers differ from nonsocial workers in their job performance and retention? If so, how? Do the same BSWs and MSWs differ from nonsocial workers in their application of social work values in their work with families and children? Are there differences between BSW/MSWs who work for public or private child welfare agencies with regards to job performance, satisfaction and retention? If so, what are they, and how can they inform us to better retain the workers we hire? Are there differences in the performances of BSWs and MSWs in child welfare? The knowledge in this area needs updating given the increased complexity of client situations.

SUMMARY

A primary task for agency-school collaborations is forging a common mission that unequivocally embraces the creating of an educated professional social work force in public child welfare. Schools and agencies must address the problem of losing sight of clients as schools become more involved in competition for students and as agencies focus more and more on winning in court, time lines and federally mandated performance outcomes. In addition, the social work profession and public child welfare agency leadership must actively endorse such a mission. Without these endorsements the ideas and recommendations contained with these special issues will fall by the wayside, continue to be our rhetoric but not our action, and/or be piecemeal efforts that do not have broad effectiveness and impact.

REFERENCES

Abramczyk, L.W., Raymond, F.B., & Barbell, I. (1992). Collaboration: The best interests. In K.H. Briar, V.H. Hansen, & N. Harris (Eds.) *New Partnerships* (pp. 81-99). The National Public Training Symposium. Florida International University, Miami, FL.

Alwon, F.J., & Reitz, A.L. (2000). Empty chairs. *Children's Voice (November)*, 35-37.

American Public Welfare Association. (1997). *Voluntary cooperative information system*. Washington, DC: Author.

Arizona Supreme Court, State Foster Care Review Board (1987). *1987 report and recommendations*. Phoenix, AZ: Author.

Booz-Allen, A.H. (1987). *The Maryland social work services job analysis and personal qualifications study*. Silver Spring, MD: NASW.

Briar-Lawson, K. (1998). Capacity-building for family-centered services and supports. *Social Work, 43*, 539-550.

Briar-Lawson, K. (2001). Building, retaining and empowering a 21st century workforce to serve vulnerable children and families. Speech given at the Children's Action Alliance Luncheon Symposium, January 18, Phoenix, AZ.

Chase, Y. & Cahn, K. (1992). Schools of social work and child welfare agencies: Barriers and bridges to better collaboration. In K.H. Briar, V.H. Hansen, & N. Harris

(Eds.) *New Partnerships (pp. 113-125).* The National Public Training Symposium. Florida International University, Miami, FL.

Chavkin, N.F., & Brown, J.K. (2002). Preparing students for public child welfare: Evaluation issues and strategies. *Journal of Human Behavior in the Social Environment* (current issue).

Clark, S. (2002). The development and evolution of the California collaboration: The competency-based child welfare curriculum project for master's social workers. *Journal of Human Behavior in the Social Environment* (current issue).

Cloward, R.A. (1998) Letters: The decline of education for professional practice. *Social Work, 43,* 584-586.

Coleman, D., & Clark, S. (2003). Preparing for child welfare practice: Themes, a cognitive-affective model, and implications from a qualitative study. *Journal of Human Behavior in the Social Environment* 7(1/2).

Costin, L., Karger, H. & Stoesz, D. (1996). *The politics of child abuse and neglect in America.* New York, NY: Oxford Press.

Council on Social Work Education. (1998). Title V-B child welfare training program awards announced. *Partnerships for Child Welfare (February), <http://www.cswe.org/partnership/feb99.htm>.*

Council on Social Work Education. (1999). Children's bureau announces child welfare training grants. *Partnerships for Child Welfare (February), <http://www.cswe.org/partnership/feb99.htm>.*

Drake, B. & Yadama, G. (1996). A structural equation model of burnout and job exit among child protective services workers. *Social Work Research, 20*(3), 179-187.

Ellett, A.J. (2001). Child welfare self-efficacy beliefs in two states: Implications for employee retention and practice. Paper presented at the Society for Research 5th Annual Conference, Atlanta, GA.

Ellett, A.J. & Millar, K.I. (2001). A multi-state study of professional organizational culture: Implications for employee retention and child welfare practice. Paper presented at the Society for Research 5th Annual Conference, Atlanta, GA.

Fox, S.R., Miller, V.P., & Barbee, A.P. (2003). Finding and keeping child welfare workers: Effective use of title IV-E training funds. *Journal of Human Behavior in the Social Environment* 7(1/2).

Friesen, L.D. (1999). Partnership examines privatization of foster care services in Kansas. *Partnerships for Child Welfare (February), <http://www.cswe.org/partnership/feb99.htm>*

Gansle, K. & Ellett, A. (1998). Louisiana title IV-E program begins evaluation process. *Partnerships for Child Welfare (February),* Alexandria, VA: Council on Social Work Education: *<http://www.cswe.org/partnership/feb99.htm>*

General Accounting Office. (1995). *Child welfare: Complex needs strain capacity to provide services.* Letter Report, Washington, DC: Reference: Gao/HEHS-95-208 (September 26).

Gomez, M. & Harris, N. (1992). Child welfare curriculum survey. In K.H. Briar, V.H. Hansen, & N. Harris (Eds.) *New Partnerships (pp. 45-51).* The National Public Training Symposium. Florida International University, Miami, FL.

Grossman, B., & McCormick, K. (2003). Preparing social work students for interdisciplinary practice: Learnings from a curriculum development project. *Journal of Human Behavior in the Social Environment* 7(1/2).

Hansen, V.H. (1992). Attitudes toward public child welfare: A student perspective. In K.H. Briar, V.H. Hansen, & N. Harris (Eds.) *New Partnerships* (pp. 37-44). The National Public Training Symposium. Florida International University, Miami, FL.

Helfgott, K. (1991). *Staffing the child welfare agency: Recruitment and retention.* DC: Child Welfare League of America, Inc.

Horejsi, C. Gaithwait, C. & Rolando, J. (1994). A survey of threats and violence directed against child protection workers in a rural state. *Child Welfare, 73,* 173-179.

Horwitz, M. (1998). Social worker trauma: Building resilience in child protection social workers. *Smith College Studies in Social Work, 68,* 363-377.

Jones, L.P. & Okmura, A. (2000). Reprofessionalizing child welfare services. *Research in Social Work Practice, 10,* 607-621.

Jordan Institute for Families. (1999). Social worker retention. *Children's Services Practice Notes, 4(3),* <http://www.sowo.unc.edu/fcrp/Cspn/vol4_no.3. htm >.

Jordan Institute for Families. (2000). Review of recent federal laws and how they affect the way we recruit foster and adoptive parents. *Children's Services Practice Notes, 4(3),* <http://www.sowo.unc.edu/fcrp/Cspn/vol4_no.3. htm>.

Kadushin, A. (1999). The past, the present, and the future of professional social work. *Arete, 23,* 76-84.

Kravitz,S. (1992). Professional social work education and child welfare. In K.H. Briar, V.H. Hansen, & N. Harris (Eds.) *New Partnerships* (pp. 25-36). The National Public Training Symposium. Florida International University, Miami, FL.

Lawson, H.A., Anderson-Batcher, D., Petersen, N., & Barkdull, C. (2003). Design teams as learning systems for complex systems change: Evaluation data and implications of higher education. *Journal of Human Behavior in the Social Environment* 7(1/2).

Leighninger, L. & Ellett, A.J. (1998). De-professionalization in child welfare: Historical analysis and implications for social work education. Paper presented at CSWE APM, Orlando, FL. March, 1998.

Levine, E.S. & Sallee, A.L. (1999). *Child welfare: Clinical theory and practice.* Dubuque, IA: eddie bowers publishing, inc.

Lieberman, A.A., Hornby, H., & Russell, M. (1988). Analyzing the educational back grounds and work experiences of child welfare personnel: A national study. *Social Work, 33,* 485-489.

Lupton, C. & Nixon, P. (1999). *Empowering practice? A critical appraisal of the family group conference approach.* Great Britain: The Policy Press.

Mather, J. H. & Lager, P.B. (1999). *Child welfare: A unifying model of practice.* Belmont, CA: Wadsworth.

National Association of Public Child Welfare Administrators (1987). *Guidelines for a model system of protective services for abused and neglected children and their families.* Washington, DC: American Public Welfare Association.

National Association of Social Workers. (2001a, January). 72 percent work for private organizations. *NASW News, 46(1),* 8.

National Association of Social Workers. (2001b, January). Clients profiles differ by setting. *NASW News,* 46(1), 12.

National Resource Center for Child Welfare Management and Administration (1994). Program redesign report conducted for the Arizona Department of Economic Security. Phoenix, AZ: Author.

National Center on Child Abuse and Neglect. (1997). Child maltreatment 1995: Reports from the states to the national child abuse and neglect data system. Washington, DC: U.S. Department of Health and Human Services.

O'Neill, J.V. (2001, April). Golden state seeks solutions to shortage. *NASW NEWS*, *46*(4), 8.

Pecora, P., Briar, K., & Zlotnik, J. (1989). *Addressing the program and personnel crisis in child welfare.* Silver Spring, MD: NASW.

Petit, M.R. & Curtis, P.A. (1997). Child abuse and neglect: A look at the states: The CWLA stat book. Washington, DC: Child Welfare League of America.

Phillips, R., Gregory, P., & Nelson, M. (2003). Moving toward collaboration: Funding as a source of change in child welfare. *Journal of Human Behavior in the Social Environment 7*(1/2).

Pierce, L. (2003). Use of Title IV-E funding in bsw programs. *Journal of Human Behavior in the Social Environment 7*(1/2).

Prevent Child Abuse America. (1996). The relationship between parental alcohol or other drug problems and child maltreatment. *Prevent Child Abuse America Fact Sheet #14.* Chicago, Ill: September.

Risley-Curtiss, C., McMurtry, S.L., Loren, S., Gustavsson. N., Smith, E., and Faddis, R. (1997). Developing collaborative child welfare educational programs. *Public Welfare, Spring, 29-36.*

Russell, M. (1988). *1987 national study of public child welfare job requirements.* Portland: University of Southern Maine, National Child Welfare Resource Center for Management and Administration.

Scannapieco, M., Connel, K., & Grager. (2002). Do collaborations with schools of social work make a difference for the field of child welfare?: Practice, retention and curriculum. *Journal of Human Behavior in the Social Environment 7*(1/2).

U.S. Advisory Board on Child Abuse and Neglect. (1995). *A nation's shame: Fatal child abuse and neglect in the United States: Executive summary.* DC: Department of Health and Human Services, Administration for Children and Families.

U.S. Department of Health and Human Services. (1999). *Blending perspectives and building common ground: Executive summary.* DC: Author.

Vinton, L. (1999). Should advanced standing programs be abolished? Yes. *Journal of Social Work Education, 35,* 7-11.

Wattenberg, E. (1998). Center prepares Minnesota students for child welfare practice. *Partnerships in Child Welfare (August),* Alexandria, VA. Council on Social Work Education: *<http://www.cswe.org/partnership/aug98.htm>*.

Young, N. (2000). Waiting children: Parental substance abuse and children in foster care. Presentation, Phoenix, AZ (January 4).

Zlotnik, J.L. & Cornelius, L. (2000). Preparing social work students for child welfare careers: The use of Title IV-E training funds in social work education. *Journal of Baccalaureate Social Work Education, 51,* 1-14.

Zlotnik, J. L.(1997). Highlights of a 60-year history. *Partnership for Child Welfare, 5,* 3,6.

Zlotnik, J. L. (2003). The use of title V-E training funds for social work education: An historical perspective. *Journal of Human Behavior in the Social Environment 7*(1/2).

Index